The Gift of Caring

The Gift of Caring

Saving Our Parents—and Ourselves—
from the Perils of Modern Healthcare

Marcy Cottrell Houle, MS,
and Elizabeth Eckstrom,
MD, MPH, MACP

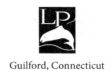

Guilford, Connecticut

An imprint of The Rowman & Littlefield Publishing Group, Inc.
4501 Forbes Blvd., Ste. 200
Lanham, MD 20706
www.rowman.com

Distributed by NATIONAL BOOK NETWORK

British Library Cataloguing in Publication Information available

Library of Congress Cataloging-in-Publication Data available

ISBN 978-1-4930-3408-6 (paperback)
ISBN 978-1-4930-3960-9 (e-book)

♾️™ The paper used in this publication meets the minimum requirements of American
National Standard for Information Sciences—Permanence of Paper for Printed Library
Materials, ANSI/NISO Z39.48-1992.

Printed in the United States of America

To my parents,
whom I loved.

To Sheri, Gladys, and Orlando,
faithful caregivers and friends.

And to John, Emily, and Jennifer,
who walked this journey with me
and proved what a precious thing is family.

To love or to have loved, that is enough.
Ask nothing further.

—Victor Hugo, *Les Miserables*

Contents

Part II: A Good Ending

Foreword

JENNIE CHIN HANSEN, FORMER CEO OF AMERICAN
GERIATRICS SOCIETY, PAST PRESIDENT OF AARP

This book is a lyrical, intimate love story of a daughter, Marcy, and how she rose and struggled to provide dignified care for each of her parents over a fourteen-year period. It's a journaling of care as she lived through the journey of their changes—with her father from Alzheimer's disease and her mother from a slow but progressive frailty. The reader travels through the struggles, triumphs, advocacy, tears, and conflicts of a devoted daughter juggling the everyday needs of herself, her understanding children, and her supportive spouse, coupled with managing a number of personal home workers from the divine to the harrowing. What makes this caregiving narrative different and special are the companion chapters written by an expert geriatrician who provides both reflection on and knowledge of what transpires in every few chapters written by Marcy.

This is a unique form of riveting narrative that gives us, as members of the general public, a useable medical understanding and practical tips that will help us anticipate, appreciate, and prepare for a more effective journey as we approach the universal care-providing experience we will all encounter— whether with our loved ones or when we ourselves will someday be given care. This book is a gift. It is written to assure the best possible dignity while also advancing the best in care as we travel the journey of life and living, until our final chapter is completed.

Preface

$\mathcal{W}$e are excited to bring you a new edition of *The Gift of Caring*, and grateful that this expanded volume will now reach a whole new audience, bringing with it even more important information to help you and your family members navigate the complexities of growing older.

For both of us, the outpouring of heartfelt response to *The Gift of Caring* has been incredible and gratifying. We have heard from so many of you—from healthcare providers, patients, caregivers, therapists, church communities, social workers, academics, students, those living in retirement communities, children with aging parents, seniors of all ages—that this book has provided you with much-needed help, plus powerful and effective tools you are using to advocate for your loved ones and yourself.

The ways you have used the information from the book are amazing:

A ninety-five-year-old woman, still very sharp, but written off by a health care provider as being "demented," was able to stand up for herself. "I am not demented," she said right back to the provider, according to her daughter. "I am just like Margaret in the book!"

A bookshop owner wrote to say her father, who had been an obstetrician and delivered over 4,000 babies, was now ninety, in a facility, and receiving dispassionate care and less-than-ideal treatment. "Thanks to your book I had the language to communicate with the staff and providers and now have a good working relationship, finally! My dad is flourishing, and now is supported. Your book gave me the necessary tools, and this is the best possible turn of events."

And then there was the physician who was given *The Gift of Caring* by her patient. "This book," she said, after reading it, "is golden."

For both of us, *The Gift of Caring* is more than a book; it is truly a mission. Perhaps one of the most rewarding things of all is that the people it has touched are now touching others' lives. With this critical information being disseminated, *The Gift of Caring* is becoming a movement! People are calling it Team Caring.

When you finish reading this book, pass it along. Share it with your own healthcare providers. Be sure your local library has a copy. Think to recommend it when friends complain about health issues or anxieties. Together we can reduce so much of the suffering that goes along with aging. Together we can improve the lives of older persons—those who have been "written off," who feel alone, hopeless, or helpless. We can improve the lives of family members caring for older parents, and can become better prepared for our own aging journey. As *The Gift of Caring* shows, aging can be so much better—for all of us.

We hope you join our Team!

Marcy Cottrell Houle, MS
Elizabeth Eckstrom, MD, MPH, MACP

I

THE AIRPLANE DIARIES

For age is opportunity no less than youth itself
though in another dress.
For as the evening twilight fades away
the sky is filled with stars
invisible by day.

—Henry Wadsworth Longfellow

• 1 •

Colliding Worlds

$\mathcal{I}$ never used to worry about getting old. Most younger people don't, but I had extra proof that aging was not a problem. You see, I was a "later in life" child; my parents had me when they were forty. My mother used to laugh that she was the oldest mother at the first grade PTA meetings. She was on the leading edge to fifty while the majority of the parents were barely in their thirties, if that.

I always thought that she had the last laugh, though, for of all my friends' parents, most considerably younger than mine, my mother and father were the most active, energetic, and fun people I knew. The word "retire" never entered their vocabulary. If he could have, my father would have continued working until the day he died. My mother did continue until she passed away, as a helpmeet to my adventuresome father and a mother of three very active girls.

My father was a doctor. Aside from my mother, the love of his life, and his family, his deepest affection was for the practice of medicine. It began when he was eight years old and visited an uncle, a surgeon, in San Francisco. At that moment, he knew that was what he wanted to be. During medical school, he refined his passion to orthopedics. There was nothing he enjoyed more, evidenced by his entreating his daughters to follow in his footsteps and all become doctors. None of us did, which he felt was a shame. The satisfaction he received from treating ailing people was deep and abiding and, in his mind, nothing could top it.

But there was more to it than just doing surgeries. His special concern was for those people who were too often cast off by society. For decades, he treated disabled children, predominantly those with cerebral palsy, and in the 1950s established the Child Development and Rehabilitation Center at Oregon Health and Sciences University, where he was a part-time professor.

3

Teaming with Shriners Hospital, the program treated disabled children from birth to twenty-one years of age. It still exists today. After spending twenty years with these patients, my father often developed a close association with them and their families.

Another segment of society was too often neglected, he thought. Through the years I saw him pay special attention to older adults. In his era, when most people turned eighty and broke their hips, a surgeon wouldn't touch them. Too risky. But my father said he firmly believed that if these old people could safely be fixed with an artificial hip and be relieved of severe pain and immobility for the remainder of their lives, it was worth the chance. He was successful, and his patients loved him. Many of those with repaired hips lived to be in their nineties and with a renewed quality of life.

Practicing good health habits was important to my father, and so it trickled down to all of us. Fitness was always a big part of his life. He loved to walk and believed that his patients and family should feel this way too. He encouraged everyone to stay active; it didn't matter how old they were. In this, he was a little bit of a revolutionary, being ahead of his time.

Living in Portland, Oregon, where the jogging fad first began with Adidas and Nike, my father took notice. Initially, it was not just for increased fitness. It was because of the shoes. After observing hundreds of patients in his practice, he believed that a large proportion of foot problems—bunions, hammer toes, rolled ankles—could be attributed to wearing the wrong kind of footwear. This was especially true with his older patients, many of whom were experiencing problems with walking. He talked to distributors and shoe suppliers and made a display in his waiting room of a sampling of three or four models of Adidas and Nike shoes. Before long, running shoes became one of my father's signature prescriptions for people with back, knee, and foot pain.

I always wanted to laugh when I saw the little old ladies going into Nordstrom wearing running shoes. I knew they had to be my father's patients.

Growing up, I saw other people growing old, but never my parents. In our twenties, some of my friends began to notice that their mothers and fathers were starting to slow down. A few began suffering from heart conditions in their early sixties or complained of mounting arthritis. Other parents started eliminating things they had once enjoyed, such as downhill skiing or long car trips or even going out at night.

Not mine. If anything, their sixties seemed to give them even more energy. At sixty-five my parents were taking some of the most adventuresome trips of their lives. At sixty-eight, my father took up jogging, and twice a week we would run together for three and one-half miles on a woodland trail near my parents' home. At the same time, my father began ramping up his care of old people. He had always made it a practice to visit nursing homes, but as he got older, he went even more often to volunteer his services for something he said was too often terribly neglected:

Caring for toenails.

All the time I was growing up I had heard about toenails. I found it a little disgusting, especially at dinner, but we all got the lecture. When people got old and confined, he explained, their toenails were often left uncut, and this caused a lot of problems. For if not properly cared for and trimmed, toenails grew thick and long and curled. Older people especially needed to have routine care, for long toenails also created walking difficulties and made for very painful feet. Too many nursing homes never bothered caring for people's feet.

This greatly disturbed my dad, for whatever reason, and so, for many years on days when he wasn't conducting surgeries or seeing patients, he carved out time to visit local nursing homes to trim old people's toenails. He never charged for his services.

Of course, like all families, health problems came up now and again in ours. In her seventies, my mother had a problem with dizziness, but with proper treatment and drugs when episodes hit, she weathered through. My father had a rough bout with prostate cancer at age seventy and required major surgery. But in my mind, as the years continued ticking by, these events were just part of life. Everyone had circumstances thrown at them that required dealing with. As a sort of proof of this paradigm, I observed my parents, while in their early seventies, still canoeing rivers, camping, and taking their little boat on excursions up the Columbia River. At age seventy-five my father was talking about taking a third canoe trip on the Yukon River.

With parents like that, who would think too much about aging? In my experience, I saw that if you worked hard, did service for others, had good friends, kept active, ate well, stayed trim, and kept intellectually curious, you could never grow old. Aging just went along for the ride, like a parallel universe that didn't really impact your real life very much. When it did—like when you needed new reading glasses or your hair got a little whiter—you didn't dwell on it.

There was another reason for my lack of worry: deep down, I felt secure in having a father who was a doctor. After watching him for forty years, I knew that doctors took care of elderly people conscientiously. I knew, with naïve certainty, if there ever came a time when we might need a doctor for him or my mother, medical support would be there. There would be plenty of doctors and nurses and welcoming hospitals and good prescriptions—like Nike running shoes—should my parents need them. And, if my dad someday couldn't cut his own toenails, well, there would always be someone else who cared enough to do it for him.

As the saying goes, what goes around always comes around. Right? Wrong. Terribly wrong.

And when the parallel universes of aging and life at last collided for my parents, I was probably the least prepared of all to grasp it. For it had never entered my thinking that this could happen to them.

Or when they desperately needed help, it would not be there.

• 2 •

First Decline

In my experience, the tsunami of growing older didn't happen all at once. Rather, it came in small floods, with drying-out periods in between. When we began seeing little hints that changes lay ahead, we discarded them, usually as quickly as possible.

This is a characteristic reaction, I believe; we want to refuse that there may be a serious problem for someone we love. So when the intermittent high waters begin coming, we refer to them, at least at first, as anomalies.

The first time my dad exhibited an uncharacteristic behavior, we decided that he must have had his mind on something else. I was visiting my parent's house when it happened. My father drove up, walked into the house, and seemed unsettled.

"I'm sure glad for my new friend. He helped me get home."

It was such an odd statement that it got both my mother's and my attention.

"What new friend?" asked my mother.

"The one I met on the on-ramp. I was coming home from Costco; the groceries are in the car. I got to the freeway and . . . thank goodness he was there."

"Did you have a flat tire or something?" I asked, rather perplexed myself. But if he had a flat tire, I would have expected him to call AAA.

"No. Nothing like that. I got to the freeway ramp, and, for whatever reason, I couldn't remember how to get home."

A chill went up my spine. My father could be sometimes, well, a bit absent minded if he had his mind trained on something else, but he had a good sense of direction.

"I pulled over, and it scared me for a second. But then my new friend came to the car window. He told me how to get home."

My mother looked puzzled, but my father seemed himself again. "Could you help unload the car?" he asked me.

Gladly. I wanted to move and forget the entire thing. It wasn't worth worrying about. I told myself there must be an explanation somewhere. And a good one came to mind right away. After working for fifty-five years, my father had recently retired from practicing medicine. Anyone's mental outlook could be compromised for a time when one was forced to retire, couldn't it? And he had seemed to take it especially hard.

My father didn't have much choice in the matter. His three partners had gently "nudged" him out—saying they thought it was time for him to quit. The fact that my father was seventy-seven years old and had continued to see patients fifteen years longer than most surgeons, who generally retired at age sixty-two, was of little consolation to him. When he shut the doors to his office for the last time, he said it was one of the saddest days of his life.

"I never thought this day would come. There's nothing else I'd rather do," he'd bemoaned, heartbroken. "I'm going to miss my patients."

"They're going to miss *you*," I said, feeling bad, too.

For an entire weekend my husband, John, and I helped move his furniture and the walls of medical charts he'd accumulated over the decades to his home, to store in the basement. My father continued being discouraged for a while—which was out of character for him. He was a highly positive person. My mother and I, discussing the matter, blamed his partners for being cold and looking only at the bottom line. Sure, office space was expensive. But it had been my father's practice; he had founded it and been the original partner. Couldn't they even leave him a little room?

Then, at about the same time as his mental lapse, another disturbing symptom became more evident. For the past year, my father's balance seemed less steady. It wasn't that he couldn't walk, or complained of pain, or shook, but his gait seemed to be getting worse, especially in the months after retiring. For a man who had been an avid outdoorsman all his life and only three years before could hike a twelve-mile loop in the rugged Wallowa Mountains in a day, this was a change. He noticed the decline, too, and didn't like it.

"I hate being feeble!" he exclaimed one afternoon after nearly slipping on a muddy section of trail in a park near his home. John, our daughters Emily (age seven) and Jennifer (age four), and I were hiking with him, as we regularly did.

"You're not feeble; it's tricky walking here," I replied, even though it wasn't.

"No; I'm just slowing you down. I shouldn't have come."

Jennifer reached him first. "You can walk with me, Papa," she said. He took her outstretched hand. Ever since she had been a toddler, she had loved walking outside with her grandfather.

A shot of pain over his unsteadiness and discouragement coursed through me. Damn his retirement, I thought, blaming it again. Why couldn't he just go on working forever, like he wanted to?

After that day, however, things seemed to level out. Not one to wallow, my father began a new routine—working from his "home office," which he set up in the laundry room. Although he didn't see patients, he spent hours researching and writing medical papers for journals—something he had done throughout his life. And while I didn't see him actually sending out anything or getting anything published, I rationalized he must be just in the "editing stages." Being a writer myself, I knew all about that. Even better, his work seemed to keep him happily occupied.

But before long a new flood came. This one was higher. It happened on a Wednesday.

For eight years, ever since Emily was born, my mother and I had a tradition: we had lunch together on Wednesdays. As a gift to me, my mother generously hired a babysitter for a few hours one day a week to give me a break, and we would go to lunch. Even when Emily, and then Jennifer, grew older and started kindergarten and grade school, we still continued with our weekly date. It gave us a chance to catch up and laugh and talk about things. I loved my mother, and so did everybody. She was kind, nonjudgmental, and had a knack for making things fun. Even in her late seventies, she liked to dress well, have her hair done, and go out to lunch.

On Wednesday, two weeks after my father's seventy-eighth birthday, when my mother and I were out together, I received a call on my cell phone from the housekeeper who occasionally came to my parents' home to clean. She said that the bank had just phoned for my mother and said it was important. I took down the number and handed my phone to my mother to dial.

From her face, I knew that something had happened.

"He did? You didn't? Did he say where he was going?" she asked, sounding troubled.

When she handed me back the phone, her hand was shaking.

"Daddy was just at Bank of California," she recounted. "The teller said he tried to withdraw $15,000."

"*What?*"

"She said he appeared confused. She told him that she didn't have that much money, or some sort of excuse, and that she would need prior approval. Thank goodness!"

"What did Daddy do?"

"She said he thanked her politely and wasn't angry, but that he left right away. He seemed so befuddled that she went straight to her supervisor."

"So where is he?"

We left our lunch half eaten and drove straight to the bank, which wasn't far. Then we drove around a few blocks. Finally, we saw him, about three streets away from the bank. We pulled over, and he was delighted to see us.

"George, what are you doing down here?" exclaimed my mother, from the window.

"I'm so glad to see you! I think I've lost my car." He climbed in with us.

As I drove around looking for his Pontiac, my mother questioned him. "The bank just called and said you tried to take out $15,000! Whatever for?"

My father didn't appear flustered anymore. "Oh yes, I went to the bank. I wanted to take out some money for our trip. I can't remember how much I asked for."

"We aren't going on the cruise for six months, and you asked for $15,000!"

"There's my car," he said, pointing up ahead on the left.

The conversation didn't seem to be registering with him, and for both my mother and me, nothing was making sense. My father was not a big spender and at times could even be called a penny pincher. Growing up during the Depression, money had always been hard to come by for his family. He had to work to put himself through college and even had to defer going to medical school after being accepted until he had earned enough to pay for it—by working in the hop fields of Oregon and being a bellhop in an old hotel on the Oregon coast. It was there, in Seaside, Oregon, where he had met my mother nearly fifty-eight years before. She had been vacationing at the hotel with her family, and he had carried her bags.

The $15,000 sum was fantastic, but my father didn't seem to be able to grasp what it meant.

"I'm going to drive you home," said my mother, still alarmed, getting out of my car to ride with him.

The floodwaters receded again after that, to both of our relief. There were no more "new friends" nor calls from the bank. My father's unsteady gait continued to be a problem, however. And two months before turning seventy-nine, while taking that cruise on the Mediterranean with my mother, he had slipped and fallen a few times aboard the ship. He never hurt himself, but each time he grew a bit more shaken. Then, one afternoon, when the ocean liner was putting in at one of the ports, he had his first major memory lapse.

"Where are we?" he'd asked my mother one afternoon.

She assumed, at first, he meant which port, but as my father had continued posing the same question to her with alarming agitation, she realized he really didn't know *where he was*. For the next few hours this had been startling, but by evening my father seemed to be himself again.

When they returned, my mother decided to make an appointment with a neurologist. Dr. Leonard was a longtime friend of my father's, having also worked with him professionally for years. At the first office visit, my mother discussed my father's new balance difficulties but couldn't bring herself to divulge anything else. Subsequently, Dr. Leonard ordered tests. For the follow-up appointment I went with them. Again, my mother and I debated, out of my father's hearing, whether we should tell the doctor of the mental incident that had occurred while on the cruise. It still unnerved her. We decided to tell Dr. Leonard about it, and we were glad we did, for he calmed our fears at once.

"Global amnesia," Dr. Leonard said. "Many people suffer an attack of transient forgetfulness. These episodes can be frightening and can last anywhere from thirty minutes to twelve hours. Some only experience it once; others can suffer several bouts. It may cause total disorientation for a while but usually clears up quickly with total recovery."

This was thrilling news.

"The problem with George is that he has peripheral neuropathy," explained Dr. Leonard. He went on to discuss that the condition was the reason for his progressive difficulty in walking and was related to his nervous system. There was damage to my father's nerves in his legs, said the doctor. The origin of the problem was unknown.

These diagnoses were a welcome reprieve. We knew that my dad had a few heart issues (but nothing requiring surgery) and some episodes of confusion, but Dr. Leonard primarily zeroed in on my father's unsteady gait. We took this to mean that my father's major problem was walking. Moreover, now my mother could provide a ready response to those concerned friends who were starting to ask, "How's George?"

"He has a nerve problem in his legs," she could say.

That explained everything. Peripheral neuropathy. If my father stumbled, or got disoriented, or even seemed a bit confused at times, it was all because of the *peripheral neuropathy*. It was just what my mother and I needed to make some reason out of the weird happenings we were beginning to observe. We could now compartmentalize our fears; we had a *name*. The other alternative explanation was, at this point, unthinkable.

For my father's birthday, we bought him a beautiful hand-carved wooden walking stick with an image of a bear's head on the handle. While he examined it with pleasure, I was suddenly stabbed with the realization that, for the first time in my life, he didn't receive a book as a present. He'd always been a voracious reader, yet somehow we all unspokenly knew that he wasn't reading much anymore. That same piercing feeling had assailed me a few months earlier, when I didn't get a handwritten card from him on my own birthday. For thirty years he had penned sweet notes to me on that day. I had saved them all. This year, there was none.

Peripheral neuropathy.

The walking stick was a hit, though. He loved it right away. It had a nice, rugged appearance. We said we would take him on a hike just as soon as possible. Everything would be just like it was before.

Excuses are great things to hide realities that our hearts aren't ready to accept. And even doctors—those who are also close friends—sometimes look to find excuses, too.

What I Wish I'd Known

Early Warning Signs of Dementia

Elizabeth Eckstrom, MD, MPH, MACP

*E*arly signs of dementia are some of the most frightening things a person and his or her family can experience. For this reason, one's first reaction is often denial. It is normal to have some word-finding difficulties with age, but denying more severe memory lapses like Dr. Cottrell had can mean a person suffers needlessly, or doesn't get help in a timely way. Some conditions of memory impairment are reversible; others may worsen through time. In most cases, though, when symptoms are observed and comprehensively addressed early, cognitive decline may be slowed for months or sometimes even years, and patient and family fears and concerns can be addressed in a timely way.

But how can you tell the difference from what is "normal" memory loss and when it is time for concern?

It is normal if an older person:

1. Experiences some word-finding problems and can't come up with the right word immediately. It is also common to forget names of people we know—only to remember them an hour later.
2. Requires extra time to process or understand things. The speed of our mental processing slows down as we age.
3. Can't seem to be able to "multitask" anymore. As it turns out, we've never been as good at it as we think we are, at any age. As we get older, multitasking becomes even more difficult. We need to learn to do one thing at a time.

It is time to worry if he or she:

1. Repeatedly forgets daily events, such as lunch plans, appointments, and birthdays.
2. Occasionally gets lost while driving.
3. Begins to prefer to have others speak for him.
4. Starts having more difficulty managing finances.
5. Loses interest in hobbies that he or she once enjoyed, such as gardening, reading, or woodworking.

What do you do if you begin seeing a parent or family member evincing a lot of red flags for memory loss? To begin with, it helps tremendously if you do one thing early:

Get to know your parent's physician.

For adult children, it is highly beneficial to form a relationship with your mother and father's doctor. Start early to establish a pattern of support—this will serve you well in later years. If you have never gone with your parent to one of his or her doctor's appointments, do it now. This will establish a growing trust between all of you—before any hard decisions have to be made. When symptoms become apparent, communication between you has already been initiated.

The next step is to gently share your concerns with your parent. Avoidance only makes for more anxiety for everyone. But how do you tell them you think their memory may be failing?

The most effective—and kindest—way to approach them is to simply share your observations without passing judgment. Never say, "I think your memory is terrible!" Rather, be objective. Calmly state, "I've noticed, lately, sometimes you seem to be struggling keeping track of your appointments. Do you think you are starting to have some memory problems?"

Then offer to help get an evaluation. This may seem scary, but stress that it's not as bad as it sounds. By this time, hopefully, you have already developed a relationship with your parent's doctor. An appointment for this kind of assessment, with you accompanying your parent, will thereby not seem so "significant" or threatening. The test may undeniably come across as a little strange—such as, "Can you draw a clock and put the numbers on it?"—but it shouldn't be seen as demeaning or frightening.

Lastly, educate yourself. Go straight to the Alzheimer's website (they have information on much more than just Alzheimer's disease) and learn about memory problems. As time progresses, consider finding classes you can attend about early dementia, and join a support group so that you can get to know others who are also helping family members with memory trouble. The more *you* know, the more you will be able to help your loved one.

Geriatricians have observed that the best outcomes occur in families where plans are discussed while everyone is *still healthy*. Parents then can lead the way. Children can listen and understand their desires. Communication has been formed in a time of no fear. Difficult questions can be asked and hashed out early on, such as: What will happen if one of you can't drive or needs daily care? Is there enough money saved for caregivers? Are finances in order? If something happens to one of you, will the other know enough to be able to take over managing things? What are your wishes if one of you must be moved to a care facility?

These are hard questions. But if thoughtfully deliberated *before* problems arise, a solid foundation can be built, which goes a long way in easing transitions. Unfortunately, too many people, like Marcy's family, will act just in the reverse order. They will begin thinking about the devastating issues only *after* they are already in motion.

Panic Attack

$\mathcal{T}$he birthday party was winding down. Seven little nine-year-olds dressed up as "pioneers" sat eating dessert on my parents' front patio. Emily had wanted a "Little House on the Prairie" theme for her party. All fourth-graders in Portland studied Oregon history, and as my family had a ten-acre woodland surrounding their home, it was the perfect place to hike deep into the forest, pretending it was the Oregon Trail. Now, back from their adventure, they eagerly feasted on cake and scoops of homemade ice cream doled out by my mother and me.

Several parents had stayed to help lead the "wagon train" so that no one would get lost in the forest. They were presently relaxing and chatting among themselves and with my parents, who enjoyed being a part of their grandchildren's festivities. Barb Fergusson came over with a plate of cake, holding it out for me with an amazed expression on her face.

"I didn't know your father had a helicopter," she said.

Obviously, the Oregon Trail had taken a toll on Barb's faculties. I laughed. "My dad never owned a helicopter."

"Well, your dad is over there, right now, telling Greg all about it. He said he loved to land it sometimes in your backyard."

"Impressive," Greg was saying, as I walked quickly over to my dad's side. "However did you manage, George, putting your chopper down with all the radio towers' guy wires around here?"

My father looked a bit confused by the question but, upon spying me, brightened. "And her mother flew it too!" he said, beaming. The cake was sticking in my throat, where my heart had just moved to.

"Her mother is a pilot," my dad continued. "The proudest day of my life was when she got her pilot's license."

"Your mother's a helicopter pilot too?" asked Greg, incredulously.

"Um, no. She has flown airplanes, though . . . sometimes," I replied, not wanting to embarrass my father in front of him. But Greg was being pulled over by Barb to help crank out more ice cream.

"Dad, you never had a helicopter," I whispered, but his thoughts had obviously moved from helicopters to my mom.

"The proudest moment, except when you were born," he added sweetly.

Always precise in detail, my father had an impeccable memory, augmented by his habit of writing everything down in journals over the past fifty years. He didn't do slip-ups like this. Greg was still looking amazed as he was questioning my mother. I saw her frown and head our direction.

"My proudest moment," my father repeated, reaching out both his arms toward my mother.

"What on earth are you talking about, George? I've never even ridden in a helicopter."

"He was just remembering the day you got your pilot's license," I intervened.

"Oh, well, I always hated flying," she said, and we both laughed.

I knew that was the truth; she only learned to fly for my dad. Since a young boy, my father had always been fascinated by airplanes and passionately loved to fly and in time got his private pilot's license, instrument rating, and even co-owned several airplanes. In the 1950s through 1970s, my parents flew all over—even round trip once from Portland to Cuba in 1949, the last year American pilots were allowed to land there. He needed a copilot—one who could take over flying the airplane if an emergency ever arose. Reluctantly, my mother agreed to get her license, although she never felt about flying as he did. When she did her first "solo," which she called a "terrifying experience," he was at the Hillsboro Airport with flowers and champagne and, of course, abounding pride.

"You were a good pilot," said my dad.

"Well, I guess I knew enough to keep my head and not panic."

"Never panic!" my father said.

I smiled, realizing it was a lesson that we could all use a little of right now. It had been a favorite phrase of my dad's, who was intrinsically a very gentle and calm person. He often brought it up in relation to many adventures he and my mother had shared. It was especially important if one were a pilot, he'd explained. "You can always think yourself out of a situation, if you don't fall to panic."

"Remember Texas?" asked my mom, her eyes teasing.

He did, and I knew he did for his eyes registered at the recollection. I had heard the story many times. It had been nearly twenty years ago, when both he and my mother had flown their own plane to Dallas to attend an orthopedic medical convention. While there, a young doctor from Missouri had asked whether he could go up for a ride. On a morning free of meetings, my father agreed. And he talked my mother into accompanying them.

Always a conservative pilot, my father respected the plane's instruments and the aviation weather reports and paid deference to the vagaries of weather. The morning of the flight dawned sunny and clear. But the extensive, flat plains of Texas can often make for some rough air conditions. My dad explained this to the doctor, who had never flown in a small plane before. The bumps would not be dangerous, he instructed, but likely more noticeable than in a jetliner. The eager young man understood and was keen to go.

Soon after takeoff the air currents got a bit choppy. My mother noticed the doctor running his hand through his hair. "This is normal," she said lightly, leaning forward from the seat behind him. "Isn't this scenery something? The landscape seems to go on forever."

"Put the plane down now," said the young doctor abruptly.

Observing the man's shaking hands gripping tightly to his seat, my father knew he needed to turn back. "Of course. If you wish," he said calmly.

"Now," the man replied, his voice rising. "Right now!"

At that moment, an inopportune bump rocked the little plane. My father quickly righted it. "We'll be back at the airstrip in five minutes; there's nothing to worry about," my father said, soothingly.

But the man's voice became more irrational. "I said I want you to put this thing down right now!" Suddenly, the doctor began reaching out at the controls.

"You need to calm down," said my father gravely.

"You don't get it!" the man shouted. "Either you put it down now or *I* will!"

My father knew they were on a course of disaster. The doctor began yanking at the steering column and instruments, sending the plane into a lurch.

"Do not touch the controls!" my father sternly cried. "I will put it down!" Scanning the horizon, he saw beneath them a four lane freeway, stretching north-south. Traffic seemed light. It was their only chance. The doctor was still panicking, grasping for the gear panel.

"Will you hold my hand?" asked my mother coolly, reaching forward to pat his arm. Something in her calm voice and the fact that the plane was really going down made the man release the control column.

Slowing the aircraft in a final descent and at the same time trying to make sure the doctor did not lurch for the yoke and pitch them into a crash, my father successfully landed the plane on the sprawling Texas freeway.

Amazingly, no one was hurt, but a car from behind plowed into the little Cessna airplane, taking out its left wing. The driver of the auto was also okay, but the plane was severely damaged. It didn't fly again for a long time.

"I was proud of *you* that day, George. You kept your head and saved our lives," said my mother. He looked at her so pleased that she added, "You have never panicked." She saw Greg and Barb walking over, getting ready to leave. "And you also *never* owned a helicopter," she added quickly.

Talk of flying helicopters and landing them in the backyard was soon forgotten. In my mind, I chalked it up to another anomaly. But before long, two more events occurred that I found I could not pretend away so easily. Both happened on the same day and occurred one month later . . . on my mother's eighty-second birthday.

It was a typical family festivity. We celebrated at our house, and my parents came over for the standard regalia of dinner, cake, and ice cream. Drifts of brown candle smoke wafted upward after my mother blew out the candles on her cake while Emily brought forth plates and forks, distributing them to everyone around the table. Handing a dish to my father, he looked at her quizzically.

"Where does that little girl live?" he asked my mother as Emily passed by.

"Why, she lives here! She's your *granddaughter*!" said my mother, aghast.

"Oh, yes. Yes, of course," he said, rapidly covering it up. But his eyes, which held a dazed expression that was becoming increasingly more familiar, belied for a moment that he really did know her.

But the next thing was even more out of character. And it happened that very same evening. At eleven o'clock, my mother called, just as John and I were getting ready for bed.

"I think he's getting worse. Much worse. All of a sudden," she said, appearing distressed.

"What are you talking about?"

"I had another fall."

"Oh God, Mom; are you okay? Should I come over?"

"No no, I'm all right. I just got up from bed quickly to go to the bathroom and, well, I think I must have fainted for a second. I found myself on the carpet."

"Are you sure you're all right?" I asked, alarmed.

"I'm fine; really. But Daddy, well, he completely overreacted. I've never seen him like this. He must have heard me fall out of bed and rushed over. He shouted something and then ran out of the room. I called after him that I was fine, but I could hear him in the kitchen, still yelling. He sounded so frightened, and that frightened *me*. Then he ran back to me." Her voice trailed off.

"So what happened? What about Daddy?"

"He's back to sleep now, thank God. But when he tore back in the bedroom I was just getting up off the floor. He was wildly waving his arms at me while I sat on the bed, and entreating me to take what he had in his hands—that it would help me."

She paused again, as if she were trying to figure out whether it had really happened or she was just having a bad dream.

"I don't understand. Are you certain you're okay? And what was Daddy holding?"

It took her a moment before she could answer. Her voice cracked. "A paper plate and a quart of milk."

4

Countdown to Advocacy

*W*e continued denying the inevitable for another year. In that time, I watched my mother change from being content to becoming pessimistic and depressed. My father's mobility was growing more impaired, but the larger issue was that his reasoning continued getting worse. Helplessly, I realized I was observing a tsunami in action—transforming my beloved parents from "young, active eighties" to elderly. My mother was frazzled, and my father, still warmhearted and caring, was displaying random moments where he seemed a terrible combination of an aging invalid with the mind of a child. The alterations were occurring before my eyes, and I was powerless to stop them.

Even worse, they were sometimes dangerous.

On one sunny afternoon while my mother was out, I dropped in to see my father. As usual, he was delighted by my visit and, as it was lunchtime, offered to share the lunch he was making with me. He was always generous— that had not changed. If ever I arrived at mealtime, he insisted on giving me part of his banana or half his sandwich. "I don't need a whole sandwich," he'd say, putting the other half on a plate for me.

"What are you cooking, Dad?" I asked. It had been some time since he had made a meal, although he had loved to cook. My mother didn't want him cooking anymore.

"I'm making chicken pies," he said, smiling the dear smile I loved so much but with the eyes growing steadily more vacant.

"What's that smell?" I said, suddenly aware of it. Before I had reached the kitchen, the smoke alarm was going off. My father had been baking a frozen chicken pie in the toaster oven. Unfortunately, he had forgotten to take the pie out of its cardboard package, and the box had caught fire. The toaster oven was spewing smoke and flame. I opened it and batted down the fire with a hand towel, quickly extinguishing it.

My father came up behind me with a look of despair on his face. "I'm sorry," he said.

It wasn't the first time we had averted a kitchen fire in the past year. A few months earlier, he had started to heat something in a fry pan on the stove and walked away. The smoke alarm had alerted my mother to the fire before she smelled anything. She too had successfully put it out. But that was when she had insisted my father quit cooking.

Upon talking with Dr. Leonard about the recent episodes and my father's continual decline in his balance, he referred us to another neurologist, saying it might be good to get a second opinion. That was the last time he saw my father as a patient. Only later did it come out why he couldn't treat my father anymore.

The new physician, after examining my father, was blunt and to the point.

"Your father has dementia," he said, "and has obviously had it for some time. I phoned Dr. Leonard to ask if he had noticed the loss in memory, and he admitted he had. I next asked him why he didn't write it in your father's chart. Dr. Leonard said he could not. He explained he had known your dad for over thirty years and respected him greatly. He said he was a great doctor and a very sweet man. It was just too difficult for him to disclose. That's why he referred his case to me.

"I don't know your father and can be more objective," he added.

It was the first time I had heard the word "dementia" and my dad's name uttered in the same breath. The physician "objectively" ordered more tests—this time, not focusing on my father's walking problem, but on his mind. The new physician scheduled an MRI, a carotid ultrasound, tests for B12 or other vitamin deficiencies, and exams to look for clots or small strokes, among other studies. When the results came in, he phoned me at home. He used another word for the diagnosis. This one was not only worse, it was devastating.

Alzheimer's.

Of course, after hanging up the phone, I knew that was impossible. My father? The one who could diagnose anything, fix everything? The doctor must be mistaken. My father was not only an educated professional but a man who was fit and adventuresome and who loved life . . . one who, not long ago, was trekking in the mountains and bicycling on the Oregon coast or canoeing in the Yukon Territory. Maybe my father just needed to walk more and a new pair of running shoes, like he exhorted to his patients . . . or maybe he needed a new doctor. There had to be another explanation. Not Alzheimer's.

Because that diagnosis was irreversible.

My heart was beating wildly. If I couldn't turn time around, at least I wanted to turn around the diagnosis. The doctor had to be wrong. And now he was referring us to still another neurologist, Dr. Christopher Hoffman, a physician who specialized in dementia. That fact gave me a twinge of hope. Dr. Hoffman, I knew, had at least a tangential relationship with my dad. Dr. Hoffman's father was an orthopedic surgeon who had worked with my father professionally.

Dr. Hoffman ran even more assessments. But they didn't change the diagnosis. They merely refined it.

When all the tests were back, he met with my mother and me to explain that he believed my father was indeed in a moderate stage of Alzheimer's. The good news was, unlike some sufferers, my father was not depressed. Dr. Hoffman referred to the disability as a "dementia syndrome," with no way of knowing how quickly it would progress. With my father's level of education, it might take longer than most. He said there was evidence also of some tiny strokes in the deeper parts of his brain, which affected balance and walking. Dr. Hoffman debated putting him on two drugs—one for his dementia, called Aricept, and one for his trouble walking, called Sinemet. A quandary in his mind was that the two could contraindicate each other.

After visiting with both doctors, I came away with the same gut reaction. There was only one explanation as to their diagnoses. Obviously they were missing something; neither doctor had found out yet what the real problem was. In essence, they were *both wrong*. We were at an impasse, and my father was continuing to become more debilitated.

The real impasse, of course, was something else entirely. It had nothing to do with the two specialists or even with my father.

It had to do with me.

My heart and head were at war. They were stuck in different places. My heart was rooted in *Denial*, refusing to budge. It had no intention of moving ahead along the road of the Alzheimer's trajectory.

My head, though, knew differently. It observed the road signs. It had just passed the one called *Denial*. Now, it had reached the one named *Diagnosis*. Just beyond that, there was another sign: *Acceptance*.

All three were crushing. Especially the last.

If not for one thing that was flagging me down, I may have continued listening to my heart, not my head, and going around in circles indefinitely while desperately seeking a way to get off this nightmarish one-way circuit. That issue was my mother. She, clearly, was getting physically worn out. I realized, painfully, that only by acknowledging the reality facing me and then moving forward, I might be able to save her.

With a sadness I had never before known, I came to acceptance. Once there, the next sign on the road was large and unmistakable: *Help needed.*

If I were to keep both my parents from falling ill at the same time, I realized I needed to find help and make some changes. But what kinds of changes? After doing some research, I concluded home health nurses were out of sight in cost. I next contacted the Alzheimer's Association, who gave me a listing of agencies, adding that I could try putting my own ad in the paper, as long as I remembered to get a police check. This sounded frightening. They also suggested that there were "facilities" my father could be placed in. Did I want a list of those, too?

Immediately, my whole being recoiled at the suggestion. My father wasn't at the point of being put out of his house. He loved his home! He enjoyed puttering in his garden, taking walks in the park with his family, eating out on occasion. He found delight taking pictures with a small automatic camera—a far cry from his professional filmmaking days, when he had produced and filmed some medical documentaries, but so what? He attempted to write in his journal. Through it all, he remained polite and appreciative.

But, I reminded myself, it was not my father, but my *mother* I was more worried about. How could I help her?

The answer came in the most unlikely of places.

At her hairdresser's.

"Mrs. Powell died," said Mrs. MacAfee, prosaically, with the objectivity about death that comes from being ninety yourself. My mother was having her hair done and was seated in a chair next to Mrs. MacAfee. The little salon near my parents' home was a kind of senior gathering place for friends since they all seemed to go to the same hairdresser, Tina, who took special care of her aging clients.

"She was a nice lady and I'm sorry. I did her hair for years," said Tina.

I wanted to smile at the scene of all the eighty- and ninety-year-olds who came to socialize and have their hair done by Tina at Cedar Crest Salon. All were adorable, whether white-haired, "natural blonde," or purple-coifed, and Tina, with her heart of gold, kept them looking that way as well as watching out for them, even phoning their sons or daughters if they didn't arrive right in time to take their mothers home. I was there on schedule.

"I'm sorry, too, about Mrs. Powell; I knew her—distantly," said my mother. "She lived in that beautiful, big house on Portland Ridge. What about Mr. Powell?"

"Dead," said Mrs. MacAfee, turning the page of her magazine.

"Mrs. Powell lived a long time; I think she was ninety-six," offered Tina. "She was so well cared for by Inez and Alonzo."

"Who are Inez and Alonzo?" I interjected, my ears perking up.

"Her caregivers," Tina replied. "Inez didn't drive, but Alonzo did. They were lovely."

"I remember that Alonzo," said Mrs. MacAfee. "He always wore a little black cap, a beret. They were from San Salvador, I believe. An older couple. He loved to cook."

"How can I get in touch with them?" I pressed, not realizing how bold I must sound.

Tina understood, without letting on her comprehension. "Mrs. Powell has a daughter who sometimes came with her. I think I may have her number."

My mother, her face reflected in the mirror, was looking at me with a slight frown. She had made it clear, many times, that she didn't need help. She could take care of Daddy just fine by herself.

Tina, though, slipped me the number when we left. By that afternoon I had contacted Inez. She and her husband were available to help. We arranged that tomorrow, at three, they would come to meet my mother and father.

There was just one snag. I had to convince my parents.

What Is Dementia, Mild Cognitive Impairment, and Alzheimer's Disease . . . and How Do You Tell the Difference?

ELIZABETH ECKSTROM, MD, MPH, MACP

So what is dementia? How is it diagnosed, and is it the same thing as Alzheimer's disease?

Dementia is a neurodegenerative disorder that gradually leads to cognitive loss and impaired function. Neurodegeneration means that brain cells become abnormal and can no longer keep your thinking on track. Five key areas in the brain are affected by dementia. Understanding them can help define the kind of dementia a person may be experiencing, for not all dementias are Alzheimer's disease. Further, in several types of dementia, ill effects and memory loss can be slowed down by implementing important changes to one's lifestyle (more on this later).

The five brain centers that are affected by dementia are:

1. ***Recent memory.*** This is the part of the brain that helps a person learn new things and remember recent events, such as what one ate for breakfast or where he put down his car keys. It also allows one to learn new skills—for example, mastering a computer program or remembering how to operate a new appliance. This part of the brain is always affected in Alzheimer's disease but not necessarily in other types of dementia.

2. ***Executive function.*** This is the area that gives a person the ability to plan or carry out a complex task. It is necessary to organize a trip, keep up with and manage finances, or follow a recipe. When this area is affected, one may begin to get lost while driving, fall behind on paying bills, or forget to add ingredients to meals, making them taste terrible.

3. ***Abstraction.*** This region gives a person reasoning ability and the capacity to see the "gray" in the "black and white" of things. If it's

26

lost, one can't see the other person's side of the story or provide accurate judgment in a time of crisis. For example, a person may notice that something on the stove has caught fire but think he can extinguish it with the kitchen throw rug rather than calling 911.

4. ***Visual spatial ability***. The brain controls the eyes, and if this part isn't working properly, one can begin having vision difficulties. They may not be able to look down, or may see blank spots, or even get left and right reversed, which can be very dangerous when driving.

5. ***Verbal fluency.*** Lots of people have mild word-finding difficulties, such as forgetting names. But people with dementia will have more severe language problems and often lose the capacity to put sentences together or understand when others speak.

Having a little forgetfulness and having to keep lots of lists does not mean dementia, as long as one is able to do everything one needs to throughout the day—even if it takes a little longer. Doctors often refer to this pre-dementia condition as *mild cognitive impairment*, or MCI. People who have MCI do not always go on to develop dementia, but many do, on average in about seven years. A few people, however, will revert back to normal.

True dementia takes many forms and is diagnosed if a person has at least two regions of the brain that are affected to the point that they are actually impacting one's function. The good news is that people with both MCI and many kinds of dementia can take steps to help prevent their memory from getting worse. These will be explained later.

Alzheimer's disease (also called Alzheimer's dementia) affects at least half of all people who have dementia. It is characterized by neuro-degeneration in the part of the brain that controls memory loss (see point 1) *plus* one other region, such as language skills (point 5) or planning skills (point 2). While the decline in function is continual in someone with Alzheimer's, changes are gradual, sometimes taking years before a person becomes severely impaired. Symptoms transition in stages, from early or mild, to middle, and late. In the mild stage, people can usually still take care of themselves but often need help with complex tasks such as finances and driving. They are still relatively strong and can exercise, participate in many activities, and enjoy time with family and friends. While people in the mild stage may forget recent events and have trouble finding the right words, they can still understand conversation and can contribute meaningfully.

As Alzheimer's disease moves to the middle stage, many patients can no longer live independently. They need help with meals, shopping, finances, driving, and other things that don't allow them to live alone. They may start to forget more important matters and lack understanding of their environment. They may also begin having trouble with activities of daily living, such as bathing themselves and using the toilet independently. In this stage, it is very important to provide structure every day so that each person can have the highest level of independence possible. Getting outside help can have immeasurable benefits and protects the health of a family caregiver, usually a spouse, who looks after the one with Alzheimer's.

When finally diagnosed, Dr. Cottrell was in the middle stage of Alzheimer's dementia. While he still could function somewhat independently, it was harder and harder for his family to explain changes they didn't know how to accept or manage.

5

A New Way of Seeing

$\mathcal{T}$hey began on a "trial" basis. They ended up staying with my parents for nine years.

"We want our privacy," my mother intoned when I told her that Inez and Alonzo were heading over to discuss spending a few hours each day with my father so that my mother could get a little time away. She was skeptical.

The privacy deal was both humorous and sad. Understandably, to have some new people in their home—possibly spending many hours a week— would be different. But as it was, right now my mother was worrying so much over my father that she spent most of her waking hours tending to him. She had cut her social life in two, and most of it consisted of what she did with my family and me. Always an outgoing, warm person who loved people, she was getting, I thought, way too much privacy these days.

Privacy had become separation from life. Soon that separation would become isolation. I didn't like the pattern I was seeing. And what would happen when my father died?

The liveliness, intelligence, and sincerity of Inez and Alonzo helped change all that. From the moment of meeting them, I knew I had struck pay dirt. Inez was a semiretired professor of Spanish at Portland State University. Alonzo had worked as a cook, chauffeur, and home aide for the past twenty years. After escaping from the revolution in El Salvador in 1980, they had found refuge in the United States and become citizens and raised their family here. They had many relatives in the vicinity, were engaging, and, on Alonzo's part, hated nursing homes, where both had worked for a stint when first arriving in America.

"I would do anything in my power to keep someone I cared for out of that," he said many times. "In our culture, we take care of each other."

I wasn't really thinking about nursing homes, but I needed something that could keep my parents safe and occupy my dad's time. We had tried, a few times, the "elder day-care" route—having my father spend a few hours at a place that catered to people with dementia—but that was a total failure for him. He didn't know where he was, wanted to be home, and spent the entire time searching for my mother. My mother and I agreed he was better off at home.

Almost immediately, Inez engaged my father and got him doing projects. Alonzo mostly showed up only to drop her off and drive her home. She came for a few hours each day, and my mother began looking forward to it and was able to plan a schedule around it. She began going out with friends again, and even a few times took a short trip to the beach or to visit my sister in Santa Fe. Alonzo and Inez stayed overnight then. Those brief sorties didn't work very well for my father, however; he couldn't understand where she was and fretted. When my mother was out of town, I had to spend most of my time with him, and Emily and Jennifer came over after school. John came by after work. Our presence seemed to relax his fears.

While my father continued to know me as time progressed, he sometimes forgot who his granddaughters were, and even John, until they identified who they were, setting things in order. In fact, it became routine for Emily and Jennifer, upon greeting him, to merely say when they kissed him hello, "Hi, Papa; it's Emily!" He always brightened then.

It had been a transition for them, too, through the past five years—observing the grandfather they loved become younger and younger in his mind, as they began getting older. Yet as we spent so much time together, the change was not as dramatic, perhaps, or as hard to swallow as for the other grandchildren, who saw him only once or twice a year. It was more difficult for them to be with him as time went on. He didn't know them, really, and they didn't know him anymore. They still loved each other, but time spent together became rarer.

This was not the case for Emily and Jennifer. We were the family who still lived in town, and, as a family, we lived through the great transition together, which meant more joy and also more sadness. Yet, on the positive side, it gave Emily and Jennifer empathy and revealed to all of us more ways to connect than I ever imagined. One of the greatest bonds, we discovered, was the time we spent in nature together.

My father's love of the outdoors did not diminish over time, even while all his other capacities did. Emily and Jennifer still enjoyed taking walks in the park when they could with their grandfather. Jennifer noticed the difference in him right away.

"He's better there, Mommy," she said. "He seems to know who we are more then, and he seems happier."

Jennifer was right. Although my father now shuffled more, needed to use a real cane on the trails built for the handicapped, and took advantage of every bench along the way to rest, he did calm down and took pleasure in the beauty of the natural surroundings. My father had been a staunch conservationist and had passionately loved his state of Oregon. Now its native landscape seemed to have some healing properties to give back to him.

On inclement days, my father stayed inside. That was when Inez's projects became invaluable in keeping him occupied. She had us purchase construction paper, crayons and colored pencils, and lined notebooks that first-graders use to learn how to write. On the tablets, she had my father practice writing his name, the names of his children, and what the date was. She asked me to retrieve and bring over all the puzzles from our attic that Emily and Jennifer had played with when they were little. Soon, my parents' kitchen became more like the one we had at home, where our refrigerator and upper walls displayed the children's artwork they brought home from school. So it was at my parents'—but there, the creations were what my father was producing. I tried not to dwell on the fact that his designs more closely resembled what Emily and Jennifer had made when they were in preschool.

However, as much as I attempted to overlook the stark incongruity that assailed me like a punch each time I visited my parents' house—trying, as we all did, to go with the flow—occasional moments still came as devastating bursts of grief. This afternoon was one of those.

Inez, as usual, had been coloring pictures with my father when I stopped by to briefly check in. She asked whether I knew where there might be a photograph of the boat he used to have, to show him and perhaps have him try to draw a rendering.

"The boat is called the *Summer*?" she asked my father, trying to get him to recollect it further.

It was, I knew immediately, the *Sumarlee*. That was the boat my father had owned since I was nine years old. For years we had cruised in it as a family every summer on the west coast of Vancouver Island. The vessel was an old air-sea rescue boat that had long ago been converted. The faithful ship was nearly as much a member of the family as any of us were. When boating had become too difficult for him to do anymore, a decade or so ago, my father made the decision not to sell it but to donate it to the Portland Sea Scouts for them to use and care for.

A thought came to mind that perhaps my father would like to see the painting he had done of the *Sumarlee* years ago. He had produced a number of oils through the years, most of them now squirreled away somewhere in the attic or basement. I went searching and found it in his darkroom next to the garage, propped up against the side wall next to the enlarger that was gathering dust. I hadn't been in the darkroom for a long time after my father quit doing photography. The room, though, was a testament to how much he loved his family. It was completely decorated with photographs he'd shot, developed, and printed of my mother, my sisters, and me, stapled on every square inch of the room's walls.

Below the painting I noticed a collection of papers, all handwritten and carefully ordered and numbered. The stack was well over an inch thick. Picking it up, I saw it even had a title, *The Airplane Diaries*, by George W. Cottrell, MD. The book came as a complete surprise; I had no idea he had been working on this before he'd gotten sick, and I wondered whether my mother knew about it. Quickly thumbing through, I saw that it was a compilation of recollections and reflections on his life. It began when he saw his first airplane up close, when Charles Lindbergh landed in Portland, Oregon. My father had been a young boy and among the public that greeted him. From that moment, my dad had been hooked on flight. The collection went on to recount many of his adventures. Clutching the pages, I forgot about the painting and ran upstairs.

"Dad, when did you write this?" I asked, holding it out to him. His eyes did not register.

"What's that?" he said, smiling and taking it.

"You wrote a book!" I exclaimed.

"I wrote a book?" he said, sweetly, not examining it, and then handed the pages back to me. He returned to his scribbling.

For a heartbreaking moment, the contrast of who he had been and what he was now struck me in the places I was working hard to protect. I felt overwhelmed, suddenly, with grief. Then my father turned to me.

"Would you like to color with me?"

Inez held out a yellow crayon.

"Of course," I said, kissing the top of his head. "Of course."

But before I sat down, I hugged the book to my chest. *I will copy this*, I thought. Somewhere, locked inside him, *this is who he is*.

My father's head was bent over the paper, as Inez was helping him draw a sailboat. Suddenly I remembered something a professor of ecology told me when I was in graduate school. He had said that when you look at an ecosystem such as a forest community, you need to adjust your thinking. Try not to be limited by seeing it for what it is right now. You need to expand your understanding to include what the forest was like in the past, and what it could be like in the future. The place you were observing at the moment was just that—a snapshot. The real, authentic place was *the whole picture*—its past, its present, and even its future. When you look to observe, he'd said, always remember to include the whole picture in your conception. That is what gives insight to the truth.

I sat down with my yellow crayon and took a piece of paper. This book could help me to remember the whole picture.

· 6 ·

Passages

It had now been six years since my father had met his "new friend" on the freeway—the one who helped him find his way home when he was lost. During that time, we had overcome four difficult transitions in the Alzheimer's journey: denial, diagnosis, acceptance, and recognizing we needed help. But a new passage was looming ahead. More than any other, I didn't want to see it, for I knew it would change things forever.

"I can't sleep with Daddy anymore," said my mother, wearily, one afternoon. "He kicks and thrashes, and wakes me up all night long with questions. And he won't wear his diapers," she said, despondently.

"Why don't we move him into my old room to sleep?" I suggested. Thinking further, I offered, "And maybe we should ask Alonzo if he can spend nights here, in the room next to mine . . . just for a while."

It would not be a difficult transition. Alonzo and Inez had been increasing their hours over the past six months, sometimes staying overnight. They had offered to come more evenings if we needed them. And on nights they couldn't stay, they had a niece, Camila, who was willing to pitch in.

My mother agreed to the plan, this time without reluctance. That reaction in itself told me something: the situation was getting worse.

But while my mother found relief in the new arrangement almost immediately, my father hated it. It took him nearly two months to adjust. After spending sixty years together in the same bed, he could not understand why his wife, the one he loved above all, would not sleep with him! Night after night he would call out for her. Inez would come to his room to try and settle him.

"I don't understand, where is my wife?" he would cry, distressed and confused. "Why won't she sleep with me? Doesn't she love me anymore?"

"George, you are up at night," Inez would repeat. It was only getting my dad to think of my mother's needs that seemed to soothe him. "Margaret needs her rest. She's tired. You wouldn't want her to be sick, would you?"

"No," he would reply, slowly. "Of course not." This calmed him for a time, that is, until he forgot what had happened and began calling thirty minutes later, "Where is my wife? I want my wife!"

Eventually, he seemed to accept sleeping in a different bedroom.

Then we made a mistake, one Alonzo always blamed himself for, but it was nobody's fault. On a night off, he had his niece, Camila, come and stay. But he forgot to tell her that my dad wore Depends at night. And that evening, she turned on the electric blanket to keep him warm.

Incontinence and electric blankets go together like hairdryers and baths. They should never be allowed to touch. Wetness leaking from my father's bladder made the electric blanket start to smolder. Soon, his bedroom was filled with smoke. The smoke alarm was too far away to pick it up. My father did not wake up. He continued sleeping soundly.

Something awakened the caregiver, Camila. Later, she said she didn't know what. But she had a feeling she should go and check on my dad. In the middle of the night, she got up, walked down the hallway, and opened his door.

A blast of smoke surrounded her. Rushing over to my dad, she struggled to wake him. At first, she could not. But she continued frantically, until she at last roused him, pulling him from the bed. They both began to cough, and she led him outside to the living room, placing him in a chair. Then she ran to get my mother.

The fire department came right away and opened doors and windows and set up giant fans to disperse the smoke. The electric blanket was ruined, of course. So was the mattress, which the firefighters threw outside. They said Camila had saved my dad's life and perhaps my mother's as well. My father likely would have never woken up, and the entire house could have easily caught fire.

The following week we got a new mattress and new blankets, not electric. We also had our three-month follow-up appointment with the neurologist and told him of the event. Thoughtfully, after examining my dad, he gently advised that my father's lack of comprehension was becoming unsafe for him . . . and also for us. While we had been dragging our heels for nearly seven years hoping the day would never come, the fifth milestone was upon us: *realizing that my father would not be able to live at home much longer.*

The question now became not when, but where. After much investigation, we put my father's name on a waiting list for a highly regarded Alzheimer's facility called "Montavilla." The unit was always full, we learned, and an opening might not become available for some time. The first thing we needed to do, they said, was to bring my father on "the tour."

A week later, my mother and I accompanied him on a visit to Montavilla. My first impression was not of a nursing home or even an elder day care.

Rather, I felt as if I had just gone back to preschool.

"Ruthanne, please give the ball to Marcy," said the nurse, who had just tossed it to the woman seated next to me.

My father and I sat in a row with eight other Alzheimer's patients. It was "recreation time," and a leader—a kind nurse named Kari—was positioned in front of us. She had already learned my father's name, my mother's name, and mine and had introduced us to the group. My mother stood behind my father, observing.

"Ruthanne, Marcy is right next to you. She would like to play."

Ruthanne clutched the pink rubber ball more tightly. It was the size of a bowling ball.

"All right, Ruthanne," said Kari, with a smile. "Can you throw it back to me?"

Ruthanne remained unmoving, still pressing the orb to her chest.

"Then please pass it to Marcy."

Staring straight ahead, Ruthanne shook her head, no.

"Ruthanne, you must learn how to share. Marcy would like a turn, too."

Ruthanne squinted her eyes at me. Her right lower lid, which was very red, hung low, giving her the appearance of a witch. She frowned, which drooped the lid even lower. With more vehemence, she shook her head.

"It's okay," I mouthed to the leader, but she ignored me. "Ruthanne, would you like to give the ball to anyone else?"

Violently, Ruthanne moved her head back and forth.

"Well then, I think Marcy *really wants* the ball. And if you don't give it to her, no one will be able to play anymore. So please throw the ball to Marcy, and play nice."

Ruthanne shoved the pink sphere into my stomach. For such a thin woman, the force of her thrust was a surprising blow.

"Now let's thank Ruthanne," said the leader. I realized she was talking to me.

"Thank you, Ruthanne," I said. Kari was still looking at me, like she was expecting me to say something more. "For sharing the ball with me," I quickly added. Ruthanne curled her lip then looked down into her lap, pouting.

"Marcy, will you throw *me* the ball?" said the leader gently, when I forgot, focusing more on Ruthanne than the game. "I think we all want to play now, don't we?"

"Yeah," I said, immediately, tossing the ball back to the leader, who then gently pitched it to my dad, who sat beside me. Catching it, he threw it right back at her.

"You catch on fast, George!" said the leader.

It was true. He figured the game out quicker than I.

After a few more rounds of catch, we moved to the crafts table. Then we walked outside into a small, locked garden. After strolling and pointing out some flowers that were similar to those around our house, we came in-side to have a bite to eat at a table with Kari. When lunch was over, we had a quick tour of some of the private rooms and another visit to the crafts table.

It had only been two hours, and I was tired. And just like I had been on my first day of preschool, all I wanted was to go home.

What I Wish I'd Known

How to Find a Good Memory Facility

Elizabeth Eckstrom, MD, MPH, MACP

*Wh*y is a memory unit helpful for a person with dementia? And how could it help Dr. Cottrell? There are lots of reasons, but three are especially important to consider:

The staff at a memory unit is trained to understand and cope with all the frustrations and problems that can arise with people suffering from memory problems. Dementia patients may have difficulty with eating, bathing, using the bathroom, keeping track of items—like their glasses or hearing aids—and may also exhibit distressing behaviors such as wandering or repetitive yelling.

None of these actions is the fault of a person with dementia, of course. But it requires special training to be able to support such patients and to maintain the highest quality of life for them.

A good memory facility is set up to keep people with dementia active and healthy, engaged in meaningful things that they like to do, and to utilize their brain to keep their memory as strong as possible. Dementia patients need exercise every day to prevent falls, improve sleep, and decrease depression. A high-quality unit stresses the importance of interesting, fun fitness programs that will help one avoid many of the medical problems that can go along with dementia.

Memory units are designed to provide help with daily functions such as bathing, eating, taking pills, and toileting. Many other types of facilities, such as assisted living, generally require that you pay extra for each care need. Moreover, most other types of facilities do not have the ability to meet the heavy care needs of patients with advancing dementia.

Once you accept that your parent or loved one needs the extra help of a memory unit, how do you find the best one?

The most essential thing is this: do research early in the process. Don't wait until you think your parent can't possibly live at home any longer; that is too late and results in far greater stress and more problems. Even worse is to postpone exploring care options until there is a crisis—such as a broken hip.

But what kinds of research?

First, visit lots of places. Have lunch at each one. And while reviewing different memory units, take mental notes. Could you picture your parents living there? Yourself? Are the people friendly? Is the environment pleasing?

Look at the activities schedules. People with dementia feel insecure when left to their own devices as they quickly forget where they are, what they are doing, and sometimes even who they are. If someone with dementia is still living at home, it is nearly impossible for a spouse or family caregiver to fill every minute with activity (though Inez certainly tried!), and this is one of the reasons memory units often help people with dementia thrive. A good memory unit will have activities planned throughout the day that are fun, that encourage socialization, and that challenge each resident to remain at his or her optimal level of function. When you are looking for a facility, look at their activities programs. Do they have things your parent would enjoy? If your parent was an artist, are there art classes? If your parent played piano, do they have one? I am constantly amazed when someone who can't remember his children or maybe even his own name can play beautiful pieces he learned as a young adult.

Be sure to check the quality ratings of facilities. Each state has a website that lists all care sites that have had "deficiencies" notes. You will want to choose from places that have a good-quality track record. In addition, be sure to ask how long the director of nursing at the facility has been there. Superior places have little turnover in their top leadership.

Ask to review protocols at each unit you visit. Facilities should have set practices in place for *non-medication* management of sleep, for falls prevention, and for avoiding restraints (be sure to also look at the residents—do any of them have restraints?). In addition, ask to see their protocols for non-medication management of dementia behaviors, such as wandering or yelling.

Talking with "transition coordinators" can also be helpful. These are people whose entire job is to assist people in finding the right facility for a family member. Most of them are paid a small amount by the facility chosen, but they often have two hundred facilities or more within their area of expertise, so they can be fully unbiased in their discussions with patients and families and simply help them choose which place is best for them. Often transition coordinators will provide a list of possible facilities that meet the individual client needs, are affordable for that person, and are convenient for family members to visit. And they will even drive you around to look at them if you would like them to! Because their salary is paid by the facility, their service is free to the patient and family—and I have seen many "perfect matches" made by experienced transition coordinators. For many families, the best option is to begin investigating different facilities together, when your parents can still help choose where they might want to go. Though this may feel like an unpalatable suggestion, it can help your parents get used to the idea. Some people may want to consider early alternatives, such as moving to a continuing care retirement community (CCRC). Both parents can move while still fairly healthy to an independent living residence and be assured that they will be able to get the care they need down the line. CCRCs often have both independent living and memory units, though they are often the most expensive of the supported living choices.

Facing the realities of declining health and memory in a parent or loved one with dementia is excruciatingly painful. The work it takes to find the best care option is time-consuming. But the amount of planning and research you do early can make a huge difference in the future health, safety, and quality of life for your parent, as well as provide comfort and support for the entire family.

7

Montavilla Beginnings

The next step in the process was having my dad spend a day at Montavilla by himself. He stayed for six hours, socializing and becoming familiar with the unit, but like every other "play date" he'd been exposed to, he couldn't wait to come home.

"It's been so long since I've seen you!" he exclaimed when my mother and I came to pick him up. He got tears in his eyes at the sight of her, said he missed her terribly, and grabbed my arm like he didn't want to let me go.

The nurse from Montavilla reiterated that although he was aware of our absence during his visit, he had seemed to enjoy himself and partaking in activities with the other inmates.

—Oops, I caught my thinking. Of course, she hadn't called them inmates; they were "clients." But in my mind, that's how I thought of them, at first. What else were they if not prisoners? They were all randomly put together in a space that was locked all around. For guests to enter, we had to be admitted plus know the key code. I understood the reasoning: this "lockdown" was because Alzheimer's patients had a proclivity to wander—that's why we all routinely read in the paper about the poor grandfather who had taken off somewhere, gotten lost, and was pronounced "missing," leaving the family nearly hysterical. No one, though, ever drifted away from Montavilla.

Clients also had an inmate quality because they really had no choice whether they wanted to be here or not. They had been *placed* here. And everything about their lives was prescribed—from their private rooms, which all faced the large, common area, to the scope of their activities, to whom they were going to interact with. I was pleased that there was the one door that led "outside" to the small but pleasant garden area we'd explored previously, and the patients could open it when they wanted and head out. But by no stretch of the imagination was it a park or natural area or wilderness—the places my father loved. No, the garden was enclosed, roofed, and walled with concrete. No one was going to escape from this garden.

The other thing: there was no getting out of Montavilla for "good behavior." Once you were there, it became home, office, vacation, cruise ship, or whatever you wanted it to be.

All in all, this place was definitely not the old familiar surroundings of home. Without even speaking the words, both my mother and I worried, how could Daddy ever be happy here? And with *these people?*

For, to be perfectly honest, it wasn't just the locked premises of Montavilla that disturbed me. The people of Montavilla themselves scared me! They seemed, well, insane. Having never been exposed to dementia before my father's illness and then entering a society of people where everybody had Alzheimer's was a formidable reality.

Ruthanne, wearing the same sneer she had when we had last visited, shuffled over in her walker when we were preparing to leave and take my dad home. She observed with her droopy eye my mother conversing with the nurse in charge and my father standing next to her, holding her hand.

My parents always held hands. Ruthanne didn't like that.

Pushing her walker closer and ramming several people in the process— she was surprisingly athletic and didn't seem to need the walker at all, using it more as a weapon—she powered her way over to stare directly at my mother and father.

"Well, hello, Ruthanne," said the nurse. Ruthanne's gray hair, although brushed, stuck out straight at all angles. I found myself cringing.

"Can you say hello to Margaret and George?" said the nurse, kindly.

Ruthanne did not say hello. Rather, she stuck her tongue out at them.

Two months later, Kari phoned my mother to say that an opening had come up at the Montavilla Memory Unit, adding that another might not for possibly a long time. Suddenly, a wrenching decision arose for our entire family.

"This isn't the way I imagined it," said my mother, unhappily. "I always thought I could let him go when he didn't know me anymore."

That day had not happened yet. And it never would. My father always knew her. And his love for her never flagged in the slightest, even at the end.

Consulting with Dr. Hoffman, he said he felt my father's illness was significantly progressing and becoming too much for my mother, even with the caregivers. Reluctantly, Alonzo and Inez agreed. Caring for my father, who was increasingly confused and needful, they admitted, was taking its toll, even on them.

The choice, as much as we didn't want to admit it, was obvious. The other option was to keep my father at home and risk his burning it down or putting my mother in an early grave from living under constant stress. Without question, though, the terrible day we moved my father permanently to his new home, the Montavilla Memory Unit for Alzheimer's sufferers, was one of the saddest in my life.

For some caregivers, understandably, it is a day of pain and relief; for me and my mother, it was only pain. We had already taken his clothes and personal belongings to the center . . . decorated his private room . . . brought things from home to make *it* seem more like home, but it was all a mask. My father loved his home, had worked with a Northwest architect to build his home from the ground up, and had lived there with my mother for fifty years. It was his familiar surroundings, where he felt safe and secure and happy.

Kari greeted us warmly when we arrived at the unit, after we had practiced inputting the code and entering the locked lobby. She skillfully engaged my dad, and he responded at once to her kindness. Together we led him to his room, where he saw many of the artifacts of his past that we had placed there. The touchstones seemed to relax him, or else, perhaps, he thought he really was at home.

For the next few hours we stayed with him, sharing lunch again together, doing a puzzle, and cutting out pictures. We nodded to some of the strange people milling around. Many activities seemed to be going on, but after crafts, we went back to his "new" familiar room, which he seemed to respond well to. It was, all in all, a good introduction—better than the previous play date.

But this was not a date. This was for forever.

My mother appeared exhausted, and Kari came over, signaling that now might be a good time for us to go. My father was ready too. He put on his beret to leave with my mother.

"George, you're staying here, with us," said Kari jovially.

Gentlemanly, my father bowed to Kari but ignored her. He took my mother's hand. My mother looked at the nurse.

"We have a brand new puzzle over here we could show you," Kari continued. A small woman with gray curly hair and a sweet smile had come up to stand behind her. In her hands she held a pair of plastic, rounded scissors, having just come from the crafts table.

"Thank you, no," said my father, turning toward the door.

"How about a cookie?" Kari was obviously trying to distract him—a great tactic in working with and motivating Alzheimer's patients—but it wasn't working. He didn't want a cookie.

My mother was quick on her feet, though, and brilliantly came up with an excuse that could console my dad about her leaving him. Actually, in time, there were three pretexts that would settle him, making him accept that my mother needed to leave—for a short time.

"I'm going to the Vista Club for lunch," she said.

The Vista Club was a ladies club that my mother had belonged to for years and where she often joined friends for light meals or to play bridge. On many of our Wednesdays together, she and I went there for lunch.

"The Vista Club?" My dad smiled. "Chicken again?"

It was a standard joke between them that all the Vista Club ever served was chicken. My father still had his sense of humor.

"Yes, chicken."

"Marcy too?"

"Yes, she's coming to lunch, too. It's Wednesday, you know."

"And then you'll probably go shopping," he said, grinning.

Shopping was the second excuse that my dad could handle. I think Kari thought that was all my mother ever did, for she immediately picked up on that and, whenever my father got agitated, wandering about and seeking my mother, she or another nurse would be able to relax him by saying, "Margaret's out shopping."

"Yes, Marcy and I are going shopping after that."

He dropped my mom's hand and kissed her. I wanted to chuckle; I never had time for shopping.

"Have fun, then. Come back soon. Enjoy your chicken," he said.

Kari, seeing a window of opportunity, took my father by the elbow and gently led him over to the crafts table, where the little gray-haired lady handed him another pair of plastic, rounded scissors.

Overseeing the entire exchange, red-eyed Ruthanne rose up to stand in her walker. Plowing it forward into another woman, she maneuvered over to the crafts table.

"He'll be fine," Kari motioned to us. "Go . . . go."

We went to the car. But we did not go to lunch. Nor did we go shopping. Instead, we stared, speechless, at the large, locked door that had inextricably shut behind us.

And we wept.

Moving Day—How to Ease the Transition

Elizabeth Eckstrom, MD, MPH, MACP

There can be nothing more difficult than moving a beloved parent out of his or her home—one where that parent might have lived for decades. Now, he will be going to an unfamiliar building with many more people around than he is used to seeing. Meals will be different from his usual fare. He will be exposed to all sorts of new sounds, smells, and sights. At first, this can be intimidating or even terrifying. All at once, he will be thrust into a new daily routine—one completely unlike what he is used to. Little wonder that the first days and weeks in a new "home" can be completely overwhelming and anxiety provoking!

There are five steps, however, you can take to make the transition for your parent less stressful and help to ease the worry, fear, and sadness over this major life change.

First, before the move, bring recognizable items from home to the new facility. Ideally, if possible, it is beneficial to transfer your parent's living and bedroom furniture. If that is not feasible, be sure to decorate the living space with pictures, favorite treasures or keepsakes, and anything that is familiar before the move. Transfer your parent's clothes and personal items so that they are all ready for use. The key is to have everything in place when your parent arrives so that he or she can walk into a place that looks like home.

Next, try to schedule the move on a day when staff members are there whom your parent has already met. A couple of familiar faces will do a lot to allay the anxiety of a new location.

Third, talk to the chef about the first meals in the facility. Make certain your parent will be eating things that are familiar and tasty. Initially, meal times will be scary in a bigger environment; the comfort of good food will provide security. In addition, it can help immensely if you eat with your parent for the first meal or two. That way, you can reduce fears as well as help introduce him or her to new people and tell them your parent's story. This has multiple benefits: others at the care unit will be happy for a new friend and, with a little help from you, will reach out to your parent.

Fourth, encourage the staff to frequently repeat their own names to your parent as well as the names of the other residents. Ask them to remind your parent what is happening with kind, gentle words. For example, if your parent's memory loss is mild, your loved one will be constantly frustrated at forgetting all the new names. Staff can help with cues, such as, "the woman who likes to wear blue is Betty." If the memory loss is more severe, however, your mother or father may not know to be frustrated by forgetfulness. Instead, your parent may be frightened by seeing constantly unfamiliar faces and places. If this is the case, frequent reorientation and soothing conversation from the staff is critical to your parent's well-being.

Finally, spend time with your parent throughout the transition to a new facility. This can be the most important thing of all. Remember, *you* are the constant feature in your parent's life. You can offer your mother or father support and reassurance. Your presence will go a long way to reduce his or her fears, make the move go more smoothly, and help your parent adjust more quickly to a new home.

8

Dallas II

*L*ife in an Alzheimer's unit, at least in Montavilla, overseen by a humane staff highly skilled with dementia patients, was far from sad. In fact, after my father became more adjusted, we had many fun times, some actually hilarious. The locked room of addled people quickly became our second home. Allowing ourselves the freedom to become a part of the patients' lives was, although sounding counterintuitive, a growing experience.

Perhaps, somewhere inside, we are all a little crazy. In time, I began to lose my fear of the "inmates" and to feel at home among them; even more, I actually began to develop a real affection for many.

What changed? I came to see the Alzheimer's sufferers as *people*, not just damaged, deranged, frightening, and sad patients. And there lay a turning point in my grief.

After one month, we had a conference with the Montavilla staff to discuss my father's adjustment. We could see the results with our own eyes, of course. My mother visited every day, usually driven to the Alzheimer's unit by Alonzo, who was staying on to help my mother out. John and I also came regularly, at least three or four times a week, and often brought Emily and Jennifer.

At first it had been a shocking experience for them to see their kind and sweet grandfather in a setting where everything and everyone seemed abnormal—like madness gone viral. But once past the initial blow to their senses, they began seeing beyond the superficialities. In time, the fear of being in the memory unit disappeared, and they could see once more into the heart of the grandfather they loved.

Nurse Kari elucidated that my father was very social. He participated in every activity (she stressed the word "every," as it showed his desire to engage and have interaction . . . a good thing) and was one of the highest-functioning patients in the unit. Too, she stressed that he was always caring to all the other people, wanting to "help" them (hopefully not operate, my mother said later). Most of all, he appeared to be happy and enjoying himself, which was a great relief. As we expected, though, there were a few problems arising from his hunting about for my mother. In this quest, he sometimes became agitated. "Where is she? Where is my wife?" he would cry.

But Kari had trained all the staff well. It didn't matter whether it were day or night. They would refrain: "She's still out shopping." If my father, a frugal man, had had his wits about him, we knew he would have been gravely concerned about the expenses she must be racking up. But time has little bearing in an Alzheimer's-affected mind, which, in some ways, can be a blessing.

The other standing problem, of course, arose whenever my mother had to leave after visiting him. These times were often the worst; seeing her again, he couldn't bear to have her out of his sight. After some rough exits, she discovered a new response that would allow her to gracefully depart.

"I've got to go, George. I've got to help Marcy with the lambs."

This was preposterous. Again, it demonstrated my father's loss of reasoning power. John, a civil engineer, and I, a writer, raised sheep and with our family lived on a small farm. Each spring we would have a new crop of lambs, which required that someone be there to assist in delivery, if necessary. My mother, a true city girl, could never figure out why we desired that kind of life. Although she thought lambs were cute, never in a thousand years would she have helped birth a sheep. My father, though, accepted this excuse necessitating her leaving. He took as fact that my mother needed to be there to perform midwifery on ewes.

"Okay," he said, reluctantly, "but come back right after they're born."

Counting all the times she used that excuse, we figured my mother probably delivered close to three hundred sheep.

Before long, I started learning something I never expected from spending more time in a memory facility. While most people wouldn't believe it if they had never experienced it, life inside an Alzheimer's unit could be as exciting as a television soap opera. Even my mother quickly picked up on all the "dramas" going on. Once we learned more about the people and observed their interactions, we began referring to Montavilla as *Dallas* II. My sister from another state became hooked right away and routinely called my mother for "updates." Just like any viewer of a popular serial, she waited eagerly for the next episode.

There were many subplots and much intrigue, and several of the unit's residents soon rose to the top as stars.

"Red-eyed Ruthanne" clearly was a leading lady. Her role in the mini-series was to break up budding romances. Whenever she saw someone who looked like a couple, Ruthanne was on the alert to nix it. Maneuvering her walker adroitly, she slammed into them to break them up. But as much as she tried, she could never disengage Bob and Bev, two other residents with top billing. This infuriated her and made her even less likely to return the ball at playtime.

Bob and Bev were an adoring couple who sat, with bags packed, on a little bench on the side of the great room in the Alzheimer's unit. Bob had been an attorney, and, amazingly, my mother had even dated him once in college at the University of Oregon. Bob had developed Alzheimer's at about the same time as my father and had been at the unit for six months when my dad arrived. Bev was not Bob's real wife, of course. His own wife, who had been a good friend of my mother's, had died over a year ago from the exhaustion of caring for him.

Perhaps, we speculated, it was the pink bib that Bev always wore that first caught Bob's eye. Most of the patients in the unit only wore the pink bibs when eating, but Bev preferred keeping hers on all the time. In fact, she never took it off, although the aides would exchange it for a clean one after meals. Actually, it looked rather stylish on Bev. She wore it canted across her shoulders, like a shawl. But whatever the reason, Bob took to Bev immediately, and, in a few weeks' time, they decided they were in love and were going to elope. Apparently, the elopement must have occurred, because they were now at the train depot, waiting for the train to take them on their honeymoon.

Day after day when I would come to visit, I would see Bob and Bev sitting happily together, unspeaking, holding hands, with their little packed bags (actually Montavilla duffels for dirty clothes) alongside them. It didn't matter, I guess, that the train never seemed to arrive. They were in love and never minded the everlasting wait.

Another star of the unit was "No-No." No-No was the self-proclaimed mother of everyone and worked hard to keep them all in line. Tall, thin, eerily gaunt, with long, bony fingers that she pointed at people to reprimand them, she continually interfered with everyone's lives. Whether it was cutting out shapes at the crafts table, coloring, exercising, or playing ball, she inserted herself, sticking out her finger. Her attention was especially honed on patients who wandered aimlessly about the room. These she would follow directly behind, exclaiming "No-no-no!"

My mother and I observed that most of the patients didn't pay much attention to her, nor, I came to think, did her own children. I learned from Kari that No-No had been the mother of eleven children. Growing up, they said she continually yelled at them to try to get control. Apparently, it didn't work the first time around. She was no more successful here with her Alzheimer's roomies, but old habits die hard.

"Stella-the-Starer" spooked me a little. She rarely spoke, only gawked. She always seemed to be on the move in her four-poster, wheeled walker, where she sat perched in the middle, like a bird in a cage with coasters. Stella had a habit of going into every patient's room to rummage through their things. Her hawk-like gaze washed over everyone with scrutiny. Her role in the cast of performers, we concluded, was as soap opera detective. It made us all wonder: *What was she staring at, and why? What did she know about everyone here?* My mother found her intense ogling disturbing. My father became disconcerted because she liked to go through his clothes, looking for something. *What did she think he had hidden in his clothes?*

As with every melodrama, there is always an actor or actress who is the crowd favorite. Mine was Eleanor. Eleanor was the gentle, gray-haired woman who had reached out to my dad with the rounded scissors on his first day. Unlike No-No and Ruthanne, who were stubborn, or Bev, who was so infatuated with Bob that she never interacted with anyone, Eleanor reached out to all the patients in the unit, as well as to their visiting families. She had a soft voice, a heart-shaped face, and sky blue eyes that were always looking out for anyone who seemed to be feeling "left out." Eleanor was a nurturer.

She enjoyed crafts, and as I often drew pictures with my dad at the table, she would come over to join us. Eleanor would chat as she cut out designs from the construction paper. In a cheerful tone, she offered help to anyone who seemed struggling with the scissors, and she never forgot to ask people seated next to her, including me, how they were feeling. If anyone seemed at all upset, she would lightly pat the person's shoulder with a kind touch. It made little difference if her neighbor did not respond to her overtures or even when Ruthanne would ram her out of spite. Eleanor took everything at Montavilla with grace. And before long, like everyone else, I was in love with her.

In fact, after greeting my dad, I would often seek out Eleanor. Soon she began to recognize me and would always come over to talk. After a few visits, I found myself wondering why she was here. It seemed a shame, really. No one came to visit her. Did her family just not want to deal with her? Perhaps they lived far away?

One day I asked Kari about Eleanor and whether she really had Alzheimer's. Kari said she did. But I never believed it until one day when I was reading a story I had written to my father.

"Oh, what lovely handwriting you have," said Eleanor, looking over our shoulders. "May I join you?"

She sat down, smiling. "My father has beautiful handwriting, you know," she continued. "Oh, how I love him. He is such a wonderful man."

"I'm sure he was," I replied. My father sat back, already forgetting about the story.

"Would you like to meet him?" Eleanor asked, animatedly. She glanced up at the big clock on the wall. "His train will be arriving in an hour. I know he'd like to meet you!"

My father nodded, and said that would be lovely. Eleanor reached out for my hand and I nodded too.

Yes, Eleanor had Alzheimer's.

· 9 ·

Visiting Hours

$\mathcal{F}$inding something to "do" when you visit someone with advancing Alzheimer's who lives in a locked facility can be a problem. After so many times playing catch, cutting out pictures, putting together puzzles, or eating a meal, you are often left yearning for more . . . or, at the very least, the desire to cut short your time together. You can't really go anywhere; you can't have a real conversation; you can't even watch TV together because someone with dementia can't follow the plot and begins to wander off.

So what *can* you do?

The breakthrough for me came by accident. In fact, it dropped out of my bag.

My father was sitting at the crafts table one morning, doing nothing in particular. He'd already finished with "exercise" and lunch was still an hour away. No one was talking, but a new resident, who had been a judge, sat next to my father, ripping colored construction paper into little pieces and putting them together in a design of sorts. "Judge" seemed to have glommed on to my dad, possibly because there weren't many men in the unit. Ernie was another friend of my father's. He was a retired firefighter. Of course there was always Bob, but Bob didn't interact much with the guys—he was too busy with Bev, waiting by the railroad tracks.

Spying me, my father broke into a huge grin and waved his arm. He glanced around for my mother, but she hadn't come out yet.

"Please sit down," he said, delighted. As there were no open chairs next to him, I grabbed one from across the table next to No-No. She waved her skeletal finger at me, scowling.

My father pushed his seat back and Judge moved over, making a space. Arranging my chair, I squeezed between them, then pulled my purse through the small opening. Unzipped, some papers and a book spilled out on the floor. It was my father's story, *The Airplane Diaries*—which I had thrown into my bag earlier to have copied. Suddenly, it gave me an idea.

"Would you like me to read the book you wrote?" I asked, collecting the pages. My father didn't know what I was talking about. I began reading anyway. Right away, Judge started to listen. After a moment, Ernie did too. But my father, especially, became enthralled.

The Airplane Diaries was not just about airplanes. It was a chronicle of many of the highlights of my father's life: when he met my mother; when he went to war—as a surgeon in the outback of Australia in World War II; when his children were born; and details of many of his adventures. That day I read only two chapters (attention spans in a memory unit are short), but it gave me something fun to do when I visited and provided immense enjoyment for my father.

On another visit I read the story of his trip down the Yukon River by canoe. The following week I entertained him reading about scuba-diving adventures off Vancouver Island. Then there was flying across the country in his little single-engine Cessna, when he circled the Empire State Building (in the days when it was still possible to do that). The book also described exploits when his plane had malfunctioned, resulting in emergency landings—none as dramatic, though, as the one on the freeway in Texas.

"Story time," as my mother called it, became a touchstone for my father. Much of the recounting he did not remember, but much he did—in a way. It made him dream of doing many of the adventures again, and we took time "planning" future trips down rivers in Alaska. Plus, Ernie and Judge always would come over to listen too. On some level, they seemed to believe the stories were about them, too.

From my time at Montavilla, I began to learn that while Alzheimer's disease compromised people's behaviors, they still were individuals deserving of respect. Some were introverts, others, extroverts. There were obstinate patients, glowerers, and fear biters, but also there were nurturers. Like all people, they had good days and bad days. After a few months of spending time with them, we began to relax. We understood the importance of having minimal expectations. And that was okay.

Only one person, though, never truly felt comfortable. And for all the times he visited, he never could shed the terror he felt when entering through the heavy, locked doors.

Alonzo.

Alonzo continued to drive my mother to the memory unit several times a week. If she had had her way, she would have still come daily, but the trip was a half-hour away, part of it on busy freeway traffic, and Alonzo tried to discourage her, saying he thought it wore her out to visit so often. In part, this was true, in part, an excuse. From the beginning, Alonzo panicked each time he entered the Montavilla stage. Why he felt such fright was a little surprising, though, considering that he quickly had become Montavilla's man of the hour—a role he held without rival. In fact, it could be said that Alonzo Mendez was America's Alzheimer's Idol.

Alonzo was a short, gentlemanly man with wiry gray hair, who dressed well and always sported a jaunty cap. Perhaps it was the hat or his South American accent, but when he showed up, the inner room just got steamier.

While my mother and I spent our time with my dad, reading or quietly sitting at the crafts table, Alonzo didn't know quite what to do with himself. After the first few visits, though, his job soon became one of fighting off female admirers. The reaction of many of the patients was indeed quite remarkable, for no other visitor elicited quite the same response. Alonzo's wife, Inez, threatened that he couldn't go to Montavilla anymore, saying that all the attention might go to his head. Even the nurses remarked that Alonzo brought out sides of some of the female patients' natures that they had not before observed.

Stella-the-Starer was a typical groupie, if any Alzheimer's patient could be called typical. She actually spoke to Alonzo, something she never did to anyone else. Seeing him arrive, she rapidly wheeled herself over to pleasantly gape at him for hours. Coyly, she asked him the same question over and over. "Are you married?"

But Stella had competition. Wanda, who always clutched a toy panda to her chest, told Alonzo that she had millions of dollars secretly hidden and that if he would come with her, they could go off somewhere together and splurge. Other women (never Eleanor) paced by Alonzo repeatedly with flirtatious smiles. One heavyset patient named Anna began calling Alonzo "Casanova."

Alonzo didn't mind that so much. But it was Ruthanne who really scared him stiff.

Of all the women, Ruthanne craved Alonzo's attention most of all. She also seemed to undergo a personality change whenever he was there. The perpetual glare she wore disappeared. Shoving the other women out of her way in her quest to come closer to her object, once reaching Alonzo, she grabbed for his arm. Instantly, Alonzo recoiled, trying to get away, but there was no place in the great room where one could escape from Ruthanne. Wherever Alonzo moved, she would track him down.

Alonzo never really knew what to do when Ruthanne refused to let go of his hand. Later, he confided that the scariest part wasn't that she liked to hold his hand but that she continually stroked it. She wouldn't let him out of her grip and caressed his big, hairy paw for as long as he could stand it. Kari commented that she never saw Ruthanne so calm. It was, she said, like Ruthanne had found her knight in shining armor.

I couldn't blame Alonzo for his reaction to Montavilla. While it was actually a restorative time for us, for him it always remained a place inhabited by crazy people. He made it clear he never desired to be a rock star. He didn't like insane asylums or soap operas, and *Dallas* II, in his mind, was the worst. He said he hoped it would run only for one season and then be discontinued.

Unfortunately for us, his wish, too soon, came true.

• *10* •

The Phone Call

*W*e received word of the accident on a sunny spring afternoon at the end of May. My father had fallen in his room. He was being taken to the nearest hospital's emergency department. After a spate of x-rays, we were told he had broken his hip and would require surgery.

When an older person falls and breaks his hip, it is life changing. If that person has Alzheimer's, however, it is devastating. Why? Because, as I learned, no one knows how to deal with an Alzheimer's patient.

Observing pain in a loved one is always a terrible thing, but when that person is your parent with dementia, the feeling of helplessness can become excruciating. What's more, at least for my father, there seemed to be little in the way of adequate pain relief, and further, hospital staff didn't know what to do with him.

Western Memorial Hospital was recognizably one of Portland's leading medical centers. My father had often performed surgeries there. But, like any hospital, at times it could become crowded and short staffed, especially on weekends or holidays. Those days always seemed to be the ones we "selected" to visit the emergency room. In fact, if I had had a calendar to plan for our trips to the hospital, it could not have been more prescribed than to hit every holiday. Through the years, we had been to the ER on Easter, New Year's Day, my daughter's birthdays, my birthday, my mother's birthday, Christmas Eve, Fourth of July, and Thanksgiving. So far, we had missed Memorial Day weekend.

The broken hip took care of that.

Holiday weekends, I already knew, were *not* good times to be admitted for a serious condition. But this time we faced the worst possible scenario. This weekend, the nurses told me, all the rooms were full. For my disabled, frightened father, there was no room at the inn.

After his initial x-rays, which were terrifying procedures for him in his demented state, my father was placed in a spare conference room. As no hospital rooms were presently available, they wheeled in a bed. Unfortunately, it was the farthest room possible from the nurses' station, which created a problem.

"Generally, we like to have Alzheimer's patients directly across from the station. We like to keep an eye on them," said the charge nurse.

That made sense. In his severe pain and confusion, my father was thrashing and crying out. He didn't know where he was.

"But, as we told you," she added, "we're full up."

"So what do we do now?" I asked, feeling more undone by the minute. Prior to this intercourse I had sent my mother home, before my dad was admitted to the main hospital from the ER and taken upstairs. My mother was utterly exhausted with worry, and I was afraid that if Alonzo did not take her home, I would soon have two collapsed patients on my hands. I promised I would stay with him if she would rest. Averse to the idea, she at last reluctantly agreed.

The nurse didn't answer my question directly. "In my experience, if we don't watch them, the Alzheimer's patient with a broken hip will become agitated and try to get out of bed and fall again," she informed. "And when they fall, they hit their head on the linoleum and crack it open. I've seen it many times."

"So you're saying, since my dad is nowhere near you and the nurses' station, someone should be with him overnight—to be safe."

She replied as if reading a script. "Like I said, they always hit their head, at least on the second fall."

There was no question; I would stay.

I called John so he could take care of the girls. I phoned my mother, telling her Daddy was settling in and, to be on the cautious side, I was going to stay the night. I tried reassuring her that everything was going to be all right.

But that was an untruth. The night was terrible. Yet while rough for me, it was a thousand times worse for my dad. He was suffering, confounded, and afraid. Being short staffed, nurses came in only infrequently. They didn't seem to know what to do. All they could say was that my father was scheduled for surgery the following afternoon. When they left, he continued lying in his bed in the conference room, yelling.

In all my years growing up, I hardly ever heard him raise his voice. For such a mild-mannered man, hearing him scream made me want to shake all over with fear. My father seemed to have lost the ability to talk. He only shouted in pain, over and over again, "Ow Wow Ow!" Or "OOOOOO." Or the words that stabbed my heart, "Oh God! My GOD!"

Why was the pain control not working? Several times I ran to the nurses' station to beg for any kind of relief. They told me he was getting pain meds. They attributed his behavior to Alzheimer's.

Their apparent lack of any emotional response to my father's outcries made me think they were used to this kind of thing. But I also began to wonder whether Alzheimer's patients were often placed far from the nurses' station. I speculated that, if situated in the center of the wing, they would be too disruptive to everyone on the floor. A distant resting spot might be a better option. Perhaps that's why the head nurse said it often happened that those patients with Alzheimer's suffered a second fall and hit their heads.

To be honest, I couldn't really blame the staff, for who could possibly relish assisting a demented old man who screamed and fought their ministrations? Each time a nurse came in to take vital signs, my father reached out to grab them, yelling at them in agony and fear. They only wished to get their job done and get out of the room. Yet while these struggles ensued, I found I wanted to scream too:

"This man is *my father*! He is a great orthopedic surgeon! Now he is weak and helpless and in pain! Please, do something!" But there wasn't much they could do other than give him a little more analgesic.

As the night dragged on, I sat in the swivel conference chair next to the roll-away bed and held my father's hand. My father slept off and on; I slept hardly at all. After dozing off for twenty minutes, I was roused by a hand shaking me shortly after 3:00 a.m.

"Dear? Dear? Wake up. My name's Robert. I'm your dad's nurse. Tonight we are really short-staffed. I need your help," he said, apologetically.

"Of course," I replied, jumping up.

"I need to place this new catheter in." He held it out for me to see. "The first one, as you know, was quite painful for him, since he has had a prostatectomy. This one is designed to be more comfortable. I need you to hold the bed pan, push it between his legs, as I work to get this in."

It was the first time in my life I had ever seen my father naked. He was a proud, private, and dignified man who would never let us see him unclothed. He even made sure my mother didn't come in if he were in the bathroom. I tried to separate the vision I was seeing now from what I knew him to be. With my free hand I stroked my father's head and talked soothingly to him. Soon Robert had successfully placed the catheter, thanking me for my assistance. My father quieted down after that; for a brief time, the terrible agitation seemed to stop. Perhaps the painkillers were working. I continued petting my father's forehead and relaxed for just a moment.

Then something happened that took me entirely by surprise. My father opened his eyes and fixed them on me. But it was a gaze I was not prepared for.

Dumbfounded, I stared back. My father was looking at me! This was not the stare of dementia. His expression was remarkably cognizant. Suddenly, it took my breath away.

For the first time in years, he was *really looking at me*!

For a moment I wanted to drop to my knees, but I didn't dare. I couldn't. For in his eyes I saw a recognition that I had not seen for a long, long time. He smiled weakly, then spoke—uttering his words in a voice that I knew and loved. But it was more than that: it was *his voice before Alzheimer's*.

"My darling girl," he said, looking into my eyes with clarity.

Then he closed his eyes to sleep. Sitting back in the swivel chair, I laid my face on the bed.

I cried like a baby.

What I Wish I'd Known

Falls—A Leading Cause of Death in Older Adults and What You Can Do to Prevent Them

ELIZABETH ECKSTROM, MD, MPH, MACP

Falls are the sixth leading cause of death in people over sixty-five and the number one fatal injury for older adults. For older individuals, they are to be avoided at all costs. Unfortunately, Marcy never knew what caused her father to fall.

Falling is caused by multiple reasons, and every older adult needs a falls prevention program to ensure safety and prevent fractures and other dire consequences of falls.

A good deal of research has been done to help families and health professionals prevent falls in older people. Following the recommendations, however, requires diligence on the part of both the family and the older adult. If consistently practiced, though, the chance of falling can be significantly reduced and perhaps save your loved one's life.

Doctors have found five things that are the most helpful in preventing falls in older adults:

1. *Regular exercise.* Deterring falls requires a good exercise program to be practiced *every day*. The best exercise to prevent falls is a form of movements developed in China, known as tai chi. This gentle exercise has been shown to cut the risk of falls *in half*. Additionally, it cuts the risk of injury from falls by 50 percent. It also decreases an older person's fear of falling, which can contribute to a vicious cycle of decreased activity and a heightened risk of more falls.

Every person over the age of seventy should do tai chi at least three days per week. Many gyms and senior centers offer tai chi classes for older adults. Seniors also need to do strength training and aerobic activity several times a week. Unfortunately, walking for exercise does not appear to reduce the risk of falls. Specific balance training such as tai chi is required and essential.

2. *Vitamin D supplementation.* Current research supports the regular use of vitamin D to reduce the risk of falls. An optimal dosage is 1,000–2,000 IUs of vitamin D3 taken daily, as this helps improve gait and balance and decrease the risk of fractures.

3. *Correct glasses and footwear.* Older persons who wear bifocals are at a higher risk of falling when they go outdoors. They should have two separate pairs of glasses to be used for different activities. One pair should be for reading and one for going out. In terms of footwear, a good pair of walking shoes should be worn for outside use and another sturdy pair of walking shoes to change into for indoors. It is vitally important that seniors never go barefoot or wear slippers or socks. Research shows this can increase an older person's risk of falling tenfold!

4. *Routine assessment for low blood pressure and heart problems.* Many older adults have reduced blood pressure when they stand up. This common problem is called orthostatic hypotension, or OH, and regularly occurs with aging. OH is a major risk for falls. With OH, when an older person rises up, he or she experiences a sudden drop of blood pressure, resulting in a feeling of lightheadedness or dizziness. The person may even faint. Certain drugs can also exacerbate hypotension, or low blood pressure.

To minimize the risk of falling, a doctor should regularly test an older person's blood pressure *two times*: once while the patient is lying down and again a minute after standing up. If blood pressure drops, a physician can then evaluate blood pressure medications to ensure they are not too strong as well as review other drugs a patient is taking that may be problematic. To help reduce low blood pressure, older adults need to keep well hydrated. Sometimes they forget to drink enough and need to be reminded. Also, staying out of the sun helps prevent rapid drops in blood pressure that can induce falling.

5. *Safety at home.* Loose throw rugs, cords, dark corners, stairways without railings, poorly lit rooms, as well as many other common items in homes all increase the risk of falling. All older people should complete a "home safety checklist" on their living space and make necessary changes to ensure fall prevention.

Surgery for an Alzheimer's Patient

$\mathcal{W}$hen a patient has advanced Alzheimer's, undergoing major surgery is akin to playing poker blindfolded. At least that is what it seemed to me. Further, it was one thing to have apprehensions when everyone was on the same page. It was entirely another, however, when you had three doctors in debate over which kind of anesthesiology offered the least chance of killing the patient.

Early the next morning I was awakened by doctor number one, Dr. Campbell. Dr. Campbell introduced himself, walked across the conference room floor, and gave my father a quick reconnaissance. He explained he was the orthopedic surgeon who would be doing the repair on my father's hip.

Thankfully, my father was still resting. He was drugged up and closely swaddled in the bed sheets in an attempt to keep him from thrashing. Dr. Campbell grabbed another swivel chair like mine and sat down opposite me, with my father situated between us, like a table.

I knew I was a mess in my wrinkled clothes, my hair unbrushed and my eyes bloodshot from crying; Dr. Campbell pretended not to notice. "Your father is coming into surgery with a lot of problems," he said, going straight to his prognosis. "His chance of surviving the surgery is fair, but to be blunt, his chance of still being alive six months out is not. No one really understands how Alzheimer's interacts with other conditions, but we know it really throws in a wrench."

My father moaned softly, still asleep, and Dr. Campbell went on. "A major problem can arise in administering anesthesia to a patient who has Alzheimer's. It can carry significant interactions of its own. Sometimes folks with Alzheimer's have real difficulty waking up after surgery."

Robert, the night nurse, was standing behind the doctor, waiting to take readings of my father's vital signs. He was listening carefully and nodding in agreement with the physician's estimation. Excusing himself to squeeze around Dr. Campbell, he applied a blood pressure cuff and made his own interjection.

"I've seen Alzheimer's patients actually take an entire month to come out of the effects of general anesthesia."

Dr. Campbell scowled and continued. "That is precisely the reason I am electing to give your father a spinal, rather than general anesthesia. I want him to *wake up*."

The information was overwhelming. A hundred questions floated in my mind, but I couldn't speak the words.

"I think your father will come through the surgery all right, even considering all the complicating factors," he said, rising out of the chair and attempting to leave me a modicum of hopefulness. "His surgery is scheduled for 3:00. I will see you then." The doctor swept his glance around the conference room and turned to Robert. "Can't you people find a better room for him than this?"

Dr. Campbell was out the door before Robert could respond and before I could formulate the one question I really wanted to ask:

"*So what happens at six months?*"

Surgery times can change. Procedures can take longer than expected; complications can arise; unanticipated emergencies will always take precedence. I knew all that from being a surgeon's daughter. But I was still somewhat disappointed to learn that my father's surgery was being set back two hours and that Dr. Campbell would not be able to do it after all, as he was tied up in what was turning into a lengthy operation. Doctor number two, Dr. Mason, met me in the conference room at 2:00 to give me the news that he was now the one who would be operating on my dad.

Wearing blue surgical scrubs, Dr. Mason strode across the floor. Thin and fit, he was older than Dr. Campbell, closer to sixty, judging from his shoulder-length white hair that he wore in a thin ponytail. He apologized that he didn't have more time to talk and then, in three minutes, rattled off a laundry list of things that could go wrong, including that my father might not make it through the surgery.

It wasn't until after he left that I remembered Dr. Mason had not said anything about which anesthetic he intended to use. When the day nurse came in to check on my father, she assured me that I would have an opportunity to direct the question to the anesthesiologist at the time of my father's surgery.

John came by, bringing me a change of clothes. Alonzo arrived with my mother, who was pale. Hours dragged until 5:30, when a nurse at last came in saying that the OR had called and they were ready for surgery.

In the operating room prep area, we awaited the doctors, with my father lying unmoving, heavily sedated. Doctor number three, the anesthesiologist, opened the curtain and, after a curt greeting, said we could wait for my father during surgery in the waiting room, four doors down. I jumped straight to the punchline about what Dr. Campbell had said before doctor number three could vanish.

"Dr. Campbell is not doing the surgery," intoned the doctor.

"Yes, I know. I only want to make sure he is having a spinal. You see, my father has Alzheimer's."

"Dr. Mason and I have already discussed it. Your father is having a general anesthetic."

I was not prepared for this—not after doctor number one had adamantly insisted that a spinal was the only surefire method to ensure my father would wake up.

"I don't understand. I think you need to talk to Dr. Campbell!"

"I have conferred with Dr. Campbell," said the anesthesiologist, sounding slightly irritable. "These are Dr. Mason's wishes, and he is the one doing the surgery. Let me be perfectly frank. Your father is at very high risk. With his heart condition, placing him on his side for a spinal might finish him off. He's old, he's frail, he's demented."

My mother's mouth dropped open. A surgical nurse came to the cubicle, preparing to wheel my father's bed to the operating room. "Be assured, everyone will do his best," concluded the anesthesiologist, pivoting on his heel to head back to the OR.

Suddenly fearful she might never see him again, my mother leaned over my father's prostrate form. Closing her eyes, she gave him a final kiss. Reaching out for my hand, we stood staring together as my father disappeared through the twin doors leading to surgery.

Alonzo was waiting for us out in the hall. With a glance at my mother's stricken face, he crossed himself. "Momma mia," he gasped.

In the crowded waiting room we sat, no one talking very much. Surgery, though, took less time than expected, and in two hours Dr. Mason came to tell us the good news that my father had withstood the procedure remarkably well. He explained that after my father had spent time in recovery, he would be taken back to his room, and we could wait for him there.

Upstairs, the floor nurse informed us he would be still in the same place.

"The old conference room, eh?" John said.

"It's been a busy day," the nurse said, piqued.

At 9:30, my father at last came up to the floor. After spending some time with him, making sure he was still not "finished off," my mother let Alonzo take her home to rest. I promised I would stay one more night to be there in case he "woke up" and needed something. In his condition, he would not know how to push a button to ring for help.

There was one good thing, I decided, about the conference room. Being so far away from the action, it was quiet. Situating my chair closer to my father's bed, I checked on his breathing and then relaxed. With heavy eyes, I was just falling asleep when jolted by someone standing over us. It was Dr. Campbell, still in his surgical clothes.

"I just thought I would pay my respects to Dr. Cottrell," he said in a soft voice so as not to disturb my father. "I'm glad that things turned out well for him today."

I wasn't sure whether I was more surprised by his visit or by the fact that he called my dad "Doctor Cottrell." I realized, suddenly, I had not heard my father referred to as "doctor" for a long time.

"Your father was a great orthopedic surgeon," he continued. "I never worked with him directly, but I knew many physicians who did. He was a highly regarded surgeon as well as a good man."

Dr. Campbell turned to leave, but stopped. Turning back to face me, he added one more thing.

"Don't ever forget that."

Events spiraled rapidly the following morning, none of which I expected. At 8:00 a.m., a discharge nurse arrived, saying my father was being transferred back to Montavilla at 2:00. He would not be returning to the Alzheimer's unit; rather, he would recover at the Montavilla Nursing Home.

"Two days in the hospital seems an awfully short time when you have a broken hip and surgery," I queried. The nurse replied it might appear so, but policy was based on the dictates of insurance agencies, and it was a holiday weekend.

"He is stable enough to be moved," she said, handing me papers to sign as his healthcare representative.

I didn't know anything about insurance dictates or recovery times, but my father certainly didn't look stable to me. Putting the papers aside, I quickly made a call to his internist, who reiterated that, unfortunately, the nurse was right; there were no other options available, as my father didn't appear to have any complications developing. He said he didn't like the quick move any better than I but admitted we were between a rock and a hard spot.

"Really what you're doing is trading one skilled nursing service for another," he said, not sounding entirely convinced himself. From my positive interactions with Kari and the staff I knew at the Montavilla Alzheimer's unit, I tried to bolster some confidence I didn't feel. At least, though, Montavilla was attentive to its patients.

There wasn't much to move; my father had not been in the hospital long enough. At 2:00, the transfer happened in short order. My mother, Alonzo, and I followed behind the ambulance carrying my father back to Montavilla. Checking in, we were told by the nurse that we were lucky; similar to the busy hospital, Montavilla was "full" and they were making an exception for my dad because he was a prior patient. His new room would be in the west wing of the nursing home, at the far back—separated from the rest of the unit by a heavy double door.

The room was spacious, and after we had my father safely settled, we felt more at ease and actually slightly encouraged. He seemed better today, his pain under control. Although he didn't understand all that had transpired in the past three days, he was conversing again. That evening, when John, Emily, and Jennifer came to visit, he smiled and said he liked the "new apartment." Even my mother laughed when he made a comment about her "do"—meaning hairdo. Like mine, after three sleepless nights, her hair was bedraggled, squashed down, lying flat to the back of her head.

"George, I'm desperately in need of having it done. I'm calling Tina, my hairdresser, first thing in the morning!"

He continued to stare at her admiringly. "You always look beautiful."

After dinner, my father fell asleep, and we left for home. Although it was unlikely, I found myself hoping that my father could improve enough to rejoin the Alzheimer's unit. Perhaps staff was wrong saying that when patients broke their hips, the setback was generally permanent. But a vision came to my mind, which made everyone chuckle. Why couldn't my father get one of those four-poster wheelchair gizmos like Stella-the-Starer had? He and Stella could pal around together and go through clients' rooms and rummage. The chairs were well padded and untippable and, if they accidentally (or on purpose, like Ruthanne always did) rammed each other, it would be akin to playing bumper cars.

Alonzo, however, wasn't keen on the idea. On the nursing home wing, at last he had found some peace—liberated from the swarming, adoring Alzheimer's fans all clamoring to pet him.

The next morning we found my father weak, pale, and panting with rapid, shallow breaths.

"George, what's wrong?" my mother cried. But his incoherent response was merely to point to the ceiling, like he was seeing angels, and mutter something incomprehensible.

"I'm going to find a nurse. Something must have happened overnight," I said, alarmed.

"Why doesn't he recognize us? Do you think he had a stroke?"

Never having witnessed one, I wasn't sure. His mouth was dry, and he picked at his gums.

"I think he is dying," Alonzo whispered.

Without waiting, I rushed down the hall seeking help. Throughout the long corridor I couldn't spy a soul. Didn't they staff anybody here? Running down another wing, I at last spotted a nurse's cart outside a patient room.

"We need your help," I said, breathlessly, racing to the door, interrupting a nurse dispensing medications. "My father's really sick."

"We'll get to him when we can."

"No, you don't understand. I mean *really* sick. Someone needs to see him right now."

"I am busy with a patient."

"I think he had a stroke!" I cried, with a sense of desperation. Calmly, the nurse excused herself from the room.

"All right; where is your father?"

"In the west wing, at the end of the hall."

Together, we proceeded through the hallways to the west wing, where we continued to the very end. The nurse shoved open the double doors, separating my father's room from the rest. Once inside his door, she observed him writhing, eyes rolled back.

"Oh my God," she said. "Let me get someone." Immediately she called to page for assistance. Two aides came in directly.

"What do you have on this patient?" she queried.

"Nothing," said one. The other aide also shrugged her shoulders.

"What do you mean, *nothing*?"

"We didn't know anyone was down here," said the first.

"Who's been taking care of him, then?"

"I don't know," answered the second aide. "I don't think anybody has. Not during my shift at least. There weren't any orders."

"What do you mean there weren't any orders?" I interjected. "My father was transferred here yesterday from the hospital!"

"I'm going to call Charlotte. He doesn't look very good," said the nurse.

The head nurse, Charlotte, arrived quickly. I recognized her as the one who had checked us in yesterday afternoon. She glimpsed my father flailing his arms upward and making grunting sounds at the back of his throat.

"I'm going to call the doctor," she said. "Get the oxygen. Where are his instructions?"

"There weren't any," the aide repeated.

"Then who has been charting him?"

She shrugged. "Not us. We weren't told anyone was in the hospice room."

Charlotte faced my mother. "Is he a hospice patient?"

"No; he's not enrolled in hospice," I jumped in, seeing my mother's stricken face. "Remember, you checked us in yesterday. He was just transferred from the hospital after having had hip surgery."

Charlotte appeared perplexed but acknowledged she remembered us from the day before. Suddenly a new thought came to me.

"If you don't have any instructions, has he had his medications? All the stuff he's on for his heart and dementia?"

"And for pain?" my mother added, pitiably. "He looks like he's in lots of pain." She was as pale now as my dad.

"I'll be back with the oxygen," said Charlotte, tersely. The aides had already disappeared.

"What do you think happened since last night?" asked Alonzo, furiously. "What did they do to him?"

Glancing around the room, I sought a cup to get my dad some water. There were none. I searched the bathroom. None there, either.

Charlotte was back within minutes, lugging the oxygen machine. She placed the mask over his nose and mouth.

"Do you think he's . . . had a stroke?" asked my mother, timidly.

"Not sure," said Charlotte. "I'm waiting to hear back from the doctor."

With the supplemental oxygen, my father seemed to relax somewhat. "I'm working to get his med orders," Charlotte continued. "Hopefully they'll be here in a few hours."

"Is someone going to come in and clean him up? He seems to be in the same diaper he came in," I said, concerned over his wound care.

Charlotte removed one of the plastic adhesives of the diaper and then tore off one side of his bandage for a peek at the incision. My father yelped in pain.

"I don't understand this," she grumbled. Looking around, she saw no bandages or diapers or any health-related materials. Next she poked her head out the door and walked into the main hall. Apparently no staff was visible for she quickly came back.

"I'm going to find someone," she said, abruptly departing.

Five minutes later, a cart banged through the double doors. I could hear the voice of an aide speaking rapidly.

"But nobody knew he was here!" the aide was appealing, defending herself. "There weren't any orders!"

Dr. Mason exploded when he heard about it. I had placed a call for him myself.

"God damn it!" he shouted. "I assumed that your father would be here at least through the weekend; that's why I hadn't written any discharge orders.

Nobody in his right mind would ship him out the day after surgery. Damn the holidays. Damn those insurance companies!"

There were a whole lot of things I wanted to damn right now. Basically, after putting together the pieces, we learned that my father had slipped through the cracks. Apparently, his broken hip had occurred *at an inconvenient time.*

There were apologies, of course. But never again, I vowed, would I let someone I loved transfer somewhere without following it up. Whether that transfer was from a hospital to a skilled nursing center . . . or from a care center to a hospital . . . or from a nursing facility to home . . . or from home to the moon and back . . . I would nevermore assume anything. Before they got to where they were headed, I would make absolutely sure their orders got there *first.* Better yet, I would hold a copy of them in my fist.

Later, Charlotte said slip-ups like this happened more often than one might expect. And not just to patients with Alzheimer's. My father was not an anomaly.

She mentioned something else too, in passing. When you're old, complications can rapidly set in. When you're old, there never *is* a convenient time.

• *12* •

It's a Matter of Life or Death

$\mathcal{T}$here was little improvement over the next week apart from the staff's realization that a patient actually resided at the end of the hall. My father's internist, in consultation with Charlotte, decided not much would be gained by rushing my father back to the hospital. Some of my father's vital signs appeared to be stabilizing—at least by the numbers that the aides recorded.

But not every disturbing symptom was abating. In fact, the most distressing ones appeared to be growing worse. My father was still in a complete fog. My mother visited him daily, but he failed to recognize her. His ability to speak had not returned. And he continued to pick at his gums—over and over again—always muttering something we couldn't understand.

Other things troubled me, too. Often when I came, I found him unclean and unshaven. His Depends were invariably wet and soiled. Alonzo noted, too, when he would visit, that my father's fingernails were dirty and unclipped, with black under them.

"That can only be from one thing," he said, angrily, "from his fiddling with his dirty diapers. Why don't they take care of him?"

Before the week was out, I knew I was on the "naughty list," because I always seemed to be complaining. Yet when I took worries to the head nurse, Charlotte, she would become concerned too. Each time she looked into a problem, she found my grievance had validity. She admitted that my father was *not* being bathed. Staff confessed they were so busy with patients that they often didn't get around to changing his Depends. Charlotte promised me that this oversight would change. But as she was rarely on the west wing, care did not seem to be improving much for my father.

I wondered about the treatment of the other patients. Rarely, I saw visitors. Charlotte said that the very sick were housed in the west wing, and I could only speculate whether their needs were being met or not. Most looked like crumpled-up, stationary lumps wrapped in cocoons of white bed sheets.

With some fright, I realized that my father, too, was beginning to resemble the rest. He was growing weaker, his tongue thicker and whiter, his cracked lips unremedied by the salve we applied. My mother called to say the nurses were commending him, however, for being "nice and quiet."

Something was wrong. Ever since returning to Montavilla, my father was a changed man. The aides attributed the symptoms to Alzheimer's. Yet somehow, the scenario wasn't adding up.

"What you need, Daddy, is *you*," I said to his unresponsive form one afternoon early in the second week. That awful swelling at the back of my throat was coming over me again. It was a mixture of terror, sadness, and even revulsion. His breath now smelled stale. His skin was dry to the touch. He seemed to be transforming into a cadaver before my eyes. Was Alonzo right? Is this what death looked like?

My father, with his eyes closed, began picking at his gums again. They were starting to bleed. That eerie grunt crackled at the far back of his throat. Reaching for the lip ointment, I dotted some around his caked mouth.

"You were always a master at diagnosing problems . . . even those that had nothing to do with broken bones," I said, suddenly feeling guilty I had not become a doctor, as he had always wanted me to be. Then, perhaps I could have helped him. As it was, a profound feeling of helplessness swept through my soul. "What is *wrong* with you? If only you could speak! You could come up with the correct diagnosis when no one else—even the internists—could. So how would you diagnose yourself?"

How stupid, I realized: entreating a semiconscious Alzheimer's victim to give me the one answer I desperately sought! With a kiss to his forehead, I picked up my purse to leave. Upon exiting, I saw his wrinkled medical chart in the box just outside the door.

"I don't know what all this means," I said, sadly. "I'm not you."

I stepped one foot into the hall and then stopped. Catching my breath, I stared back at the chart. An idea had jumped into my head.

"But maybe I can *play* you."

No aide was in sight, as usual. And wasn't I his healthcare representative? Perhaps I should ask a nurse whether I could take a peek at his chart.

Forget that. They would only resist, probably citing HIPAA. Well, forget HIPAA too. Without a second thought, I grabbed up my father's chart and began reading.

It was pathetically thin, with nothing that I didn't know aside from one or two words. Snatching a pen from my purse, I wrote them down. Then I scanned his drug list. Most of them I recognized already: Aricept for his dementia, Sinemet for his partial Parkinson's symptoms, some medicines for his heart and cholesterol. There were one or two new things, though. Perhaps something he was allergic to. I wrote the drugs down.

I replaced the chart into its container. Stuffing my notes in my purse, I went to the car. For another idea had come to me. I had an hour.

And I knew just where to go.

"There's nothing here I can see that would result in the symptoms you are describing," said Phil, after reviewing my list. He discerned the disappointment in my face. "I can go over the side effects of each one if you'd like, but your dad has been on most of these medications before."

Phil was the pharmacist at our local drugstore and had known my family for a long time. Each time I went in for something, he asked about my father. I knew he wouldn't consider me crazy for asking for his help.

"No, thanks anyway," I replied. "It was just a wild hope."

"In fact, there's only one new drug on this list since we last dispensed his medications here." The pharmacist pointed his finger at the page. "Lasix."

"What's that for?"

"Lasix is prescribed to help prevent congestive heart failure, to keep fluid from filling up the lungs. It draws water from the tissues."

Phil stopped short.

"*Dehydration*," he stated.

"What?"

"Of course. *That* could explain your father's dry mouth, slurred speech, and overwhelming weakness. Dr. Cottrell may well be severely dehydrated if he is on Lasix and the nurses aren't pushing lots of fluids."

I thought back to the lunch trays. I couldn't remember seeing any drinking glasses on them. In fact, I had never yet seen the aides give him fluids.

"I think you'd better call the doctor," said Phil.

The internist immediately ordered blood work to evaluate my father's sodium and chloride levels. Both tests came back alarmingly high, proving that my dad was indeed extremely dehydrated. Lasix was discontinued at once and a unit of fluids prescribed. The doctor explained to the Montavilla nurses about my father's serious condition and instructed them to make sure he had plenty to drink.

My entire family could not thank Phil enough for saving my father's life, but the pharmacist humbly waved off the praise. What he said in passing, though, probably saved my father's life a second time, although we didn't know it then.

"Just a piece of advice," he added, thoughtfully. "If I were you, I would ask the nurses to chart his intake of liquids. You know, to be on the safe side."

"No," they responded flatly at my request when I asked them. "We are not a hospital. Charting fluid intake is out of our purview."

When I told Phil their reply, he shuddered.

"God, I don't want to ever turn eighty. Please keep me out of the hospital or the nursing home. As a pharmacist, you hear the stories . . ."

My father's doctor asked for a repeat blood draw later in the week to re-check my father's electrolyte levels and kidney function, after the infusion of a unit of fluids. Unfortunately, this test, too, confirmed that my father's sodium and chloride levels were still dramatically elevated. He called one evening with the bad news while I was preparing dinner.

"The results show your father's kidneys are failing," the internist informed. "I'm very sorry. It is the explanation for the abnormally high readings. Right now it's only a matter of time."

"Matter of time? Until he dies?"

The doctor was consoling but realistic. "Right now, your father cannot process the liquids though his kidneys. We tried giving him a unit of fluids with instructions to keep him hydrated. Unfortunately, his kidneys are shutting down."

"But how can you be sure?" I entreated. "What if it's because he is not getting enough fluids at the nursing home?"

"For these kinds of results, Montavilla would have to be giving him practically no fluids at all," said the doctor. "My advice is to get your family together. There is nothing more we can do. If you're a praying type, all you can do now is pray."

Dropping the phone into its receiver, I sank down into the chair. From the kitchen window John's headlights appeared as he drove into the garage. Emily was practicing piano. Jennifer was caught up with some tricky math problems for school tomorrow. Dazed and cold, my body felt as if someone had just poured icewater down my back. I waited for the tears to come.

But they did not. For I realized, there *was* something I could do— besides praying. There was still one last thing . . . something the pharmacist told me to do.

The nurses might refuse to chart my father's fluid intake, but that didn't mean that we couldn't. We could be there at every meal, throughout the day, to make sure my father was getting something to drink.

I reflected again on those guttural utterances escaping from my father's throat. I could not let my father die and wonder whether they weren't really desperate cries:

"*I am thirsty.*"

A Deadly Fate with Few Symptoms— Dehydration—How to Recognize It and How to Prevent It

Elizabeth Eckstrom, MD, MPH, MACP

*W*ater is a basis of human life. Of a person's total body weight, 60–70 percent is water. For bodily systems to properly function, water plays an essential role. It is a necessary component for carrying critical nutrients to body cells. It helps regulate the body's temperature. It moves oxygen to cells throughout the body. It is fundamental to the liver and in flushing out waste products from the kidneys. It plays a principal role in lubricating joints.

Without water, the body cannot perform its tasks. Without adequate hydration, the body will shut down and die.

In frail older adults, dehydration is the most common cause of fluid and electrolyte disorders. Once these set in, other problems can quickly follow. Dehydration can cause confusion, weaken the immune system so that infections more easily take hold, and even slow the healing of bedsores.

Dehydration is ranked as one of Medicare's top ten admitting diagnoses. Persons between the ages of eighty-five and ninety-nine are six times more likely to be hospitalized for dehydration than younger individuals. It is especially harmful in senior citizens, becoming life-threatening more rapidly and causing organ failure, for they have less reserve to fight it.

Prevention of dehydration should be a primary concern when one is caring for older individuals, and the ability to recognize the early signs and symptoms can be critical.

What happens when people become dehydrated?

When fluids aren't replaced in the body, a person's total blood volume is decreased. A fluid loss of just 1–2 percent of body weight begins to compromise heart, body temperature regulation, and muscle function. For example, heart rate rises an additional three to five beats per minute for every 1 percent of body water loss. If the dehydration continues, the lack of blood volume and weakened pumping efficiency of the heart lead to diminished blood to the brain, the liver, and the kidneys. Eventually, multiple organ failure will result.

Why is dehydration such a problem in older adults?

Older people are at greater risk for dehydration by virtue of the aging process itself. While there are numerous reasons, six are foremost:

1. Loss of muscle. As people age, they lose their lean body mass, or muscle, and increase their proportion of body fat. While muscle can contain 73 percent water, fat is nearly free of it. This equates to less water throughout their bodies. Older people's water content is 60 percent—approximately 10 percent less than that of the younger population. This puts older people at a higher risk of dehydration.

2. Diminished capacity to thermoregulate. Older persons are more prone to temperature-related health issues. They have a much narrower range of safe temperatures that may vary no more than 2 degrees from the normal temperature of 98.6 degrees Fahrenheit. For older people, when body temperatures dip below 96.6 degrees or above 100.6 degrees, problems may result. Their ability to sweat and shiver is dramatically reduced, for their thermoregulation functions do not work as well. Even slight increases in ambient temperature can be difficult for older individuals. When the weather gets hotter, they require 10 percent more to drink to help keep them from overheating. Limiting caffeine and alcohol, staying indoors during the heat of the day, and the generous use of cooling fans or air conditioners all can help maintain a frail person's temperature regulation. Dehydration of greater than 3 percent of body weight increases the risk of developing heat illness (heat cramps, heat exhaustion, heat stroke). Heat illness is common in older people and can occur after just one hour of activity in the heat.

3. Infection. Many infections can lead to dehydration, and this often happens quickly in an older adult. There are several reasons infection can cause dehydration. Fever is one of the most important—a fever causes sweating and lots of fluid loss. Older persons with a high fever need rapid medical assessment and fluid replacement. Having an increased rate of breathing also causes more fluid loss, so infections like pneumonia often lead to dehydration. Other causes of shortness of breath such as heart problems can also lead to dehydration. Urinary infections can cause increased urination and lead to dehydration.

4. *Medications, including diuretic therapy.* Many medications that older patients take for age-related diseases such as high blood pressure and congestive heart failure put patients at increased risk for dehydration. Older people who take these medications often need extremely careful blood volume control and should weigh themselves (or be weighed) regularly to keep their fluid status normal.

5. *Inability to recognize when they are dehydrated.* Older individuals have a decreased awareness of thirst. Even when they are dehydrated, they may not feel thirsty and forget to drink. For older individuals in good health, eating and drinking may become less of a pleasure over time because of diminishing senses of taste and smell. And older adults with cognitive impairment may not feel hungry or thirsty and forget to eat and drink for long periods unless someone else helps ensure adequate nutrition and fluids.

6. *Powerlessness to rectify dehydration themselves due to disability and lack of access.* This can be a serious problem in understaffed nursing homes. Studies have shown that dehydration affects two out of every five nursing home residents.

Because dehydration is so prevalent in older people and can have such serious ramifications, it is important to be able to recognize its symptoms before its effects become severe. Unfortunately, identifying the signs can be difficult, as many of the warning indicators can be assumed—even by trained healthcare individuals—as being normal in an older individual.

In the beginning stages, older persons may only feel a dry or sticky mouth. Their eyes may look sunken and their skin dry. They may experience dizziness or muscle weakness and have a headache.

Dizziness is a particular problem. It is caused when the decrease of fluid volume is enough to cause decreased blood pressure when standing. This "orthostatic hypotension" can create lightheadedness, which increases a person's risk of falling.

When dehydration becomes moderate, an older individual may become very thirsty. There is little urine output. Their pulse becomes more rapid, and blood pressure drops even more.

In severe cases, a patient can become delirious or even unconscious. When this happens, rapid intervention is essential. Any older person who is dehydrated should have a medical assessment to determine the cause and then safely and rapidly have the dehydration reversed. Finally, it must be ensured that dehydration does not recur.

What can I do to make sure my loved ones don't become dehydrated?

Make sure they have plenty of fluids! If the temperature outside is rising, be certain they have access to even more! It is crucial that older persons get plenty to drink and reminders to drink often, even if they don't feel thirsty. Most older adults need about six eight-ounce glasses of nonalcoholic, noncaffeinated liquid daily. Because their body needs fluids to stay healthy, provide them an assortment of beverages to choose from. Include foods in their diet that have high water content, such as fruits and vegetables, soup, and yogurt. And if they have a medical illness that requires fluid restriction (such as congestive heart failure), be sure to talk with their doctor about what to do in hot weather *before* it gets hot.

If you have concerns that your parent may be showing signs of dehydration, talk to his or her doctor. Also, chart how much fluid your loved one is taking in. If you can't do it, ask your parent's caregiver or nursing home to keep records. Well-run nursing facilities will record what a patient eats and drinks.

Dehydration is a serious condition and, for the elderly especially, it can become life-threatening. It was for Dr. Cottrell. If severe dehydration is not diagnosed early enough, the mortality rate for older adults can be as high as 50 percent! Unfortunately, in the aging population, it is common and precipitates many grave problems. The good news is that dehydration is entirely preventable. Developing an awareness of it, watching carefully for warning signals, and helping your loved ones keep their fluid levels up, especially in times of warmer weather, can have far-reaching consequences.

Remind. Replenish. Restore their fluids.
Water can save their lives.

• 13 •

Forsaken

The campaign began. Rightly or wrongly, I decided to postpone telling my mother and sisters what the doctor had said. I needed to give my father one last chance. And between John, Alonzo, Inez, and me, we worked out a plan. One of us would be with him at all times during the day and at meals douse him with fluids. My mother was not a part of the strategy; she was exhausted and growing weak herself. I worried that if she were cognizant of what we were devising, she would be at the nursing home in an instant, day in, day out. Now, her rest was more critical; if we failed in our attempts, there would still be time to say our good-byes.

From the ravenous way my father consumed each glass of cranberry juice, the cans of Ensure, the chocolate milkshakes, the Gatorade, and especially the cups of water we gave him, my hunch that he must still be severely dehydrated only grew. I began suspecting that the aides never brought him any liquids at all.

The notion was confirmed by Alonzo.

"This is the third time I've been here at lunch and there were no drinks on your father's tray!" he growled, calling me at noon on the third day of our watch. "I did as you said, complained to the aide. She said, 'The kitchen forgot.' Forgot! And in his condition!"

My time with my dad was at dinner, after John came home from work. I brought Gatorade and chocolate Ensure, which he took to voraciously. Our chart of fluid consumption was growing, as well as my anger that for the past three dinners, no fluids had arrived with his trays. Same thing at breakfast, reported Inez.

This was unconscionable. Tracking down a nurse, which took some hunting, the aide appeared unruffled. "Talk to the kitchen. Tell them to make sure they include fluids with his tray," she said.

"Isn't that something you're supposed to do?" I asked, "as his nurses?"

"We don't have time to check over what's on everyone's trays. We just feed what the kitchen gives us."

I stormed to the kitchen next. But the response I received was no better. "We just put on what we're told," one worker said.

"Who tells you?"

"The nurses."

"Well, *I'm* telling you, put on fluids!" I shouted, but my voice paled in the noise from industrial dishwashers running full steam.

I returned to my father's room demoralized. The whole thing seemed a hopeless cycle of frustration. It was a boxing match of wills, and I was losing. Even more, I felt beaten to my core. My opponent's endurance, backed by indifference, had successfully rendered me powerless to fight.

It had been ten days since my father had uttered a word. When he gulped down his cups of water, he had his eyes closed, like a zombie. We had to hold his head up to drink, or else he could choke. Not knowing what else to do, I reached for another chocolate Ensure, stashed in the little refrigerator I brought to my father's room two days earlier to house cold drinks. Greedily, he slurped the canned shake down like a desert traveler coming upon mountain spring water after days in the blazing sunshine.

On day five of the vigil, my mother called. She sounded breathless. She was visiting my father, and as I hadn't seen him for over a day—John had taken my shift—my first thought was that he must have taken a turn for the worse.

"You must come out here right away! Inez and Alonzo are here. Daddy's *changed!*" she said, screeching.

Oh God, he is dying. And no one has said his good-byes—

"He's sitting up!" she cried. "He just took a cup of water and smiled at me. He *smiled!* Then he said, '*Hi, darling!*'"

She was crying. "I'll be right there." Throwing down the phone, I ran to the car. Arriving thirty minutes later at the west wing, I found a different man.

The doctor made a third appointment to retest my father's blood chemistry. Although a little surprised by the turn of events, he didn't want to lend false hope. "When a person is dying, sometimes he can evince a burst of strength and seem better all of a sudden. But after that," he cautioned, "they return to their decline."

This wasn't just a burst of strength, I knew, feeling my father's hand holding mine. The Room at the End of the Hall was a happy place tonight. While my father didn't know exactly who we all were, he was yet smiling at everyone in the room: at my mother, who held his other hand, at John, Emily,

Jennifer, and Inez and Alonzo. There was no more gum scratching, gagging, or gesticulations with his arms.

"You're a nice girl," he said, putting my hand to his lips to kiss it. At that moment an aide walked in carrying my father's dinner.

Dropping off the platter on a bedside table, she smiled, then departed. All eyes turned swiftly to the tray. It held not a drop of fluid.

Lab tests showed exactly what I expected: my father's sodium and chloride levels were normal. His kidneys were not shutting down after all.

"Your father should recover well. He was only severely dehydrated," said the doctor.

I wrote a letter to the director of Montavilla documenting what had happened, but my mother begged me not to send it.

"What if they don't treat him well after they read it?"

"They don't treat him well now, and they need to know," I replied. But even I had some reluctance, with the same anxieties. My letter cited specific details and dates of what we had observed, including his lack of daily care—with no one on staff helping him with meals, bathing, or shaving—and drew attention to the painful bedsore he was developing on his buttocks. I had listed each time the meal trays had been served without drinks and included a copy of our own fluids chart documenting our attempt to offset this grave and life-threatening oversight.

I ended the four-page epistle with a plea:

Dr. Cottrell compassionately cared for the infirm so much during his lifetime. All I ask for is that he receive a little of the respect in his failing days as he so willingly gave to others. It is a terrible worry for our family to think that if we aren't there to watch out for him, no one at Montavilla really cares.

For several days I carried the letter around in my purse. Even Alonzo counseled that I think twice before giving it to them, fearing some retribution toward my dad. Only John and my children were adamant.

"You must give them that letter—for Papa's sake," said Emily, forthrightly.

But it wasn't until I came for a visit the following week and found my father struggling in his bed, feet bound up by twisted sheets, his expression like a frightened dog trapped in underbrush, that I made my decision. Extricating him from the bedding, I saw he was clothed only in a dirty diaper with coffee spilled all over it. My father's lunch tray sat unopened on a table across the room.

Shoving open the double doors, I hunted down Charlotte. Recounting my father's condition, she stormed through the west wing and into his room. Immediately, she called for the aide and then chewed her out. The aide cowered, and I felt a little sorry for her.

"How long has this food been sitting here?" barked Charlotte.

"I guess for a couple of hours. We've been really busy. I'm sorry. It's cold now. I'll go reheat it."

"Reheat it?" said Charlotte, disbelieving. "What do you think you're doing? That food has been sitting out for hours! Warm it up and it could give him food poisoning on top of everything else!"

Charlotte shook her head with impatience. "Just take it away," she grumbled, as the aide nervously picked up the tray. "And get someone in here to clean this patient!" The aide nodded and trotted down the hall. Charlotte continued shaking her head and faced me with remorse.

"I want you to know how sorry I am you've had to go through this. I've had it with this wing. I know how upset your family has been over your dad. Montavilla's usually—not this bad."

"Will you read something?" I asked her, taking the letter from my purse.

The nurse scanned the four pages, blanched, and handed it back. "You must show it to the director." The vehemence in her voice surprised me. "I've had serious concerns about the west wing for some time. It's terribly understaffed. Lately a lot of temps have been brought in."

She turned to me confidentially. "I think you should know something. I probably shouldn't be telling you this, but I did a little checking." Charlotte went toward the door and pulled it shut behind her. "Your father isn't the only one in trouble on the west wing."

I stared at her quizzically.

"It may all be a coincidence; I don't know. But last week, *six people died on this wing*."

No Man Is an Island

$\mathscr{W}$hen one is seeking out real estate, three words can differentiate whether a home is desirable or not. The same principle is true for nursing homes: *location, location, location*.

After my letter was received by the director of Montavilla, things rapidly changed for my father. Immediately he was transferred out of the west wing (terrible location) and situated in the main building, in a pleasant room just across the hall from the director's office (better location). No one could miss seeing him there, which meant—to our minds—he had a better chance of not being ignored. This seemed to be the case: amazingly, the unkemptness of his room, his soiled clothes, and his regularly unshaven face were quickly remedied.

Further, never again at Montavilla was a meal tray delivered to my father without a large glass of water.

Yet while his critical needs were being met, new challenges were arising. He required more care in terms of help getting in and out of a wheelchair and assistance with a litany of medications, and although he had regained much of his speech, his ability to follow a conversation, especially any instructions, was greatly diminished.

Before long, I observed that the daily routine at the nursing home was dissimilar from my father's previous residence at the Alzheimer's unit (best location), where all staff had been trained and were highly skilled in dealing with Alzheimer's disease. Here, in the main nursing home, not all patients had dementia. Rather, they evinced a myriad of maladies. Socially, they were not a "community" at all but formed loosely associated assemblages, some more isolated than others.

In an attempt to comprehend the entire experience, I began envisioning the nursing home as one giant Montavilla Sea, made up of an archipelago of islands, each with its own culture. For there were several distinct communal groups, arranged by mental and health functioning.

The most populous island was easy to pick out. It was the "Land of the Pink Bibs." Linear in configuration, this island was actually one long row of patients that every day were lined up by the nursing staff next to a wall in the hallway. Sitting side by side in their wheelchairs, these inhabitants stayed mostly in place—to be fed, checked on, or attended to when necessary. They didn't move around or talk much, but having them all in one place made it easier for the aides to feed them all at once.

Then, there was the island called "Activities Room." This was not quite as densely packed as Land of the Pink Bibs and seemed to have one or more distinct geographic regions as well. Depending on one's interests, a patient could linger at Television Bay and watch TV all day long. A few regulars did just that. Crafts didn't seem to exist in Activities Room. There was a piano at one end that no one played. There was one locale in the room, though, where the more "with it" residents seemed to congregate. This was Street of Reminiscences—where staff on occasion rounded up people and encouraged them to talk about the good old days.

Although it was above his functioning level, I tried Street of Reminiscences one day with my father. At once I could see that men were in high demand there. A few older women took note of my father. Of a large circle of thirteen, only three patients were male.

"What did you do on New Year's Eve?" asked the recreation specialist to the group. "Does anyone remember?"

My father did not have the slightest understanding of what she was talking about. Don, one of the trio of males, did, though, and responded right away.

"Kiss the girls!" he shouted.

"Thank you, Don," said the aide. I could tell that she was hoping to get other people to join in, for she cut Don off right away, turning toward the rest.

"What about any Christmas traditions? What do you remember? Are there any you'd like to share?"

"Kiss the girls!" chimed Don again.

"Thank you, Don. Ladies, I want to hear from you. What about other holidays? Thanksgiving, for instance. What did you do on Thanksgiving to celebrate?"

"Kiss the girls!" cried Don.

"Kiss the girls," my dad echoed, smiling. Don nodded. He was on a roll.

"Louise," said the aide, ignoring them both, "can you come up with another holiday?"

"Fourth of July?" said Louise, shakily.

"Good! So what did *you* do on the Fourth of July?"

"Kiss the girls!" Don blared.

"Well, we know what kind of man *you* were," said the aide, giving up.

The saddest islands, in my mind, were single atolls composed of only one patient. These residents were the castaways—left by themselves in their rooms, with various degrees of dementia or too ill to socialize. They seemed to be always alone, for I rarely saw visitors. Most of their time was spent sleeping or staring at the ceiling. More like vegetables than human beings, their prospects looked grim.

I swore my father would never share that fate. But with his deepening Alzheimer's, there didn't seem to be a lot of alternatives. After his fall, he couldn't understand TV anymore nor hold a real conversation with anyone. His friends from the Alzheimer's unit weren't allowed out of their own wing. In front of my eyes I could see the disease was robbing him of society by setting him further and further apart from others. It would not be long, I feared, until he would be just another inhabitant in the row of the Isle of the Pink Bibs.

I discussed the problem at dinner one night with my family, relaying my peculiar image of the Montavilla Sea, with its random, floating islands and isolated atolls. At first, John looked at me like I had lost my mind. But then Jennifer said something that stopped all of us short.

"Well, if you can't take Papa to the different islands like TV Land or Activities Room anymore, then why don't you *bring the islands to him?*"

She had found the answer, unlocked the secret.

Emily caught on immediately.

"Jennifer's right. We could bring Papa the Island of Music. He loves music. And they've got a piano there, too. We could play for him like we used to, when he was home."

"And the Island of Nature," Jennifer added. "I know he can't go outside anymore, which is sad, but we could bring him some pictures to look at."

More ideas were thrown out. I suggested we could wheel him to the chapel. Emily thought we should bring out our golden retriever for him to pet, if Montavilla would allow it. Then John came up with one of the best ideas of all.

"Your dad always loved family celebrations. Parties. Bring to him the Peninsula of Parties."

"How would I do that?"

"Isn't there that open room off the dining room?" John suggested. "Maybe you could throw a little party there—you know, birthday, Valentine's, or just make the reason up. I'd bet he'd enjoy it."

It was evident that all the proposals had a similar vein: they sought to touch a part of my father that was still approachable. They were directed not to his intellectual intelligence but to his emotional intelligence. This was the *intelligence of the heart.* While everything else might fail, that understanding, even for someone with Alzheimer's, did not.

But all these ideas relied on one important factor: visiting. I could already discern that, at least to a small degree, the more we routinely visited my father, the more he was able to hold on to part of his personality. While he did not always know who we were and had forgotten our names, he still knew us through his heart.

As Jennifer suggested, we brought my father islands. Music was a special favorite. It seemed to reach a deep place in him, generating a calming effect as well. We bought my father a boom box and purchased a number of CDs. Interestingly, his favorite, which he enjoyed hearing over and over, was *Mozart for Your Mind: Boost Your Brain Power with Wolfgang Amadeus.*

"Do you think I am getting smarter, too?" said my mother, hearing it for the hundredth time. "I must be."

He also enjoyed a suite of CDs called *Music for the Mozart Effect; Heal the Body.* The lyrical quality of the music lent a completely different atmosphere to the depressing room and carried all our minds and imaginations far from Montavilla to a place of satisfaction and, at times, even joy.

As Emily had noted, Montavilla had a piano in the Activities Room. Rarely was anyone in that part of the room. When they came to see him, Emily and Jennifer often played the piano for him, which my father loved. Sometimes it didn't matter what tune they played; he would break out happily singing, "I've Been Working on the Railroad."

The chapel, too, was a peaceful spot for all of us, providing a place where my father could feel some serenity and tenderness. For many of the nursing home residents, the little room seemed to give them a sense of dignity and grace far beyond the constricted life they otherwise knew at Montavilla. The chapel was lit with candles, and light streamed through colorful stained-glass windows. The stillness and tranquility of the place provided the perfect ambience for my father—to fall asleep in his wheelchair.

But when we brought Party Island to Montavilla, he woke up. To its credit, the nursing home let us take over the space off the dining area when we planned a party. Often we put up one or two decorations before wheeling him in and set up food and something to drink. These revelries allowed us to keep a shred of lightness and gaiety in our lives together at Montavilla. At the very least, it kept nursing home life from getting too boring.

And because a party for my dad wouldn't be a party without champagne, I purchased a set of plastic champagne flutes so we could toast each other—

repeatedly. Of course, because of his Alzheimer's, my father was not allowed alcohol. We improvised. We filled the glasses with sparkling cider and my father did not know the difference. But seeing the wine glasses, the nurses sometimes grew nervous. They wanted to make sure we were following the rules.

Not wanting to upset the staff or invoke the possibility of their rescinding our use of the room, I asked Charlotte one afternoon, "Would you prefer us to drop the sparkling cider, champagne thing?"

"Not at all," she replied. "A lot of patients enjoy a glass of wine here occasionally. Your father's not a problem. The one who I am worried about is Ruth."

Ruth was ninety-five and lived a few doors down. She was very sharp still and, as Charlotte explained, had no alcohol restrictions.

"So what's wrong with Ruth?"

"I'm afraid she may be nipping the bottle a bit *too* much," Charlotte confided. "Two weeks ago, her son brought her a half-gallon container of Bailey's Irish Cream as a gift. In less than a week, an aide found it half gone. Yesterday, the same aide said she couldn't locate the bottle at all. I asked Ruth about it. Ruth said she'd finished it! When I asked her how she possibly could have consumed a half-gallon of Bailey's in one week, she responded, 'Honey, living here, I'd lose my mind if it weren't for liquor!'"

In time, I came to see that all of the activities we brought provided us two essential things. First, they gave us something to do when we visited, which became as important for us as for my father. Having a plan provided impetus to keep coming regularly—requiring us to be creative, which kept things from getting too sad.

But it also allowed us something that would not have happened if we had visited only rarely. Spending time with him kept our connection with him *alive*. It gave us the opportunity to continue *seeing the whole person through Alzheimer's*.

And some of the occasions were especially tender. One such evening in particular, which I always cherished, was a celebration of a real event: my parents' sixty-first wedding anniversary.

John, the girls, and I met Alonzo and my mother at Montavilla, bringing dinner and almond "champagne." As my mother had been fighting a nasty cold, she had not been out to visit for several days. My father, seeing her again after the weeklong absence, was at first so moved he could not speak.

Reaching for her hand, his eyes filled up with tears, which, of course, made all of us tear up too. He stared at her devotedly, as if he had not beheld her face in years.

"You are so beautiful!" he exclaimed, unwilling to release her hand.

My mother was obviously embarrassed. "Happy anniversary," she said.
"You are so beautiful," he said again. "Are you *married?*"
"Yes," she said, smiling. "I'm married to you!"
"To me? You are?" My father closed his eyes, then opened them again.
"*To me!*" he said, in adoration. Taking her hand to his lips, he kissed it.
Then he laughed and laughed with joy.

What I Wish I'd Known

Communicating with Those Who Have Alzheimer's Disease or Other Dementias

Elizabeth Eckstrom, MD, MPH, MACP

If you are a family member or caregiver for someone with Alzheimer's disease or another type of dementia, you have probably struggled to have a good conversation with them. Moreover, as memory problems progress, meaningful communication seems to grow more difficult.

At these times it is important to be mindful that, more than words, "conversations" can be opportunities to be in the moment with them, to find a new level of closeness, and to connect in new ways. Communicating with someone with dementia is multifaceted, with a larger goal of offering comfort, attempting to ease anxiety, and letting a person know he or she has value. Learning what to anticipate as dementia advances, as well as techniques you can use to help preserve a person's self-identity, can allow you ways to connect with your loved one.

So what can you expect? Early in the course of the disease, persons with growing cognitive impairment may ask repetitive questions, forget parts of a conversation within a few minutes, and have trouble comprehending complex stories or conversation with emotional content. This is because they are experiencing diminished abstract reasoning ability. At this stage of the disease, communication should focus on using simple language. It helps to speak in short sentences and not to try to communicate too many things all at once. And since decisions become more difficult and stressful, saying, "I have made you a delicious turkey sandwich for lunch," will often work better than saying, "what would you like for lunch?"

Your loved one will still be able to respond to single questions. They can remember clear, short stories if repeated several times, and will likely be able to tell detailed stories about things that happened in the past. This is a great time to ask your family member to tell lots of stories of their past. It's an activity that can be fun for both of you and you may learn things you never knew before! The key is to be sure to give them plenty of time to tell their stories. Don't finish sentences for them or try to assist with word retrieval unless they ask for help. If they don't remember, move on to a different subject. It can be upsetting when they see they can't please you by simply recalling what you are asking.

As dementia progresses, many people have diminishing language skills. They can no longer complete a sentence and cannot understand even simple stories or instructions. This is the time to watch for "good days." Some people with moderate and advanced dementia will spend several days or weeks without speaking much, but then have a day when they can tell a story or seem to understand when they are listening to you talk.

These are the days to relish. It is your chance to see your loved one the way they used to be. For most days, however, it becomes necessary to connect with your loved one with advancing dementia without being able to have a full conversation with them.

But how do you do that? From working with patients with Alzheimer's for many years, I have found several methods that aid in the ongoing struggle with communication. Seven stand out in maintaining connection and providing a sense of well-being for your loved one.

1. Even if your loved one is not talking with you, don't stop talking with them!

Tell them what is happening in your day, what successes any children have had at school, news of family and friends, even what the weather is like. Your loved one may understand more than you realize, and will enjoy hearing your conversation, even if it seems they don't recognize what you have said.

While a person with dementia may no longer understand your conversation, hearing you speak will give them joy and provide a sense of security. After all, your voice is familiar to them—they have been listening to you talk for many years! If you are a new non-family caregiver for a person with dementia, frequent conversation using a gentle tone will help establish familiarity and trust.

2. Listen to what your loved one is saying and maintain eye contact during conversations—even if they are not forming sentences as well as they used to.

It is important to give your loved one time to complete their thoughts. Be patient and prepared for this. Also, encourage them to keep trying to finish what they are attempting to say, rather than—what we are prone to do—quickly taking over the conversation.

The Alzheimer's Association has more communication tips about this at their website: https://www.alz.org/national/documents/brochure_communication.pdf.

3. When language is less effective for connecting, try music.

When Dr. Cottrell had difficulty communicating, Jennifer and Emily discovered what would work for their grandfather—music. We all have deep emotional ties to music (who hasn't enjoyed belting out "I've been working on the railroad?") that are stored in different parts of the brain than our language center. These are often reachable long past the time our language is accessible to us.

It is not surprising for someone with advanced dementia who cannot talk to be able to sing, or even to play the piano or another instrument they have played all their life. I advise looking into a great program called MUSIC AND MEMORY (musicandmemory.org) that has been developed for dementia care homes. It uses stored memories of music, often best-loved and familiar songs, to help calm sadness or other distressing emotions of those with dementia.

The underlying theory of MUSIC AND MEMORY is that cognitive impairment, or memory loss, leads to a reduced ability to process sensory stimuli. In turn, this can mean a person with dementia will experience increasing levels of stress, resulting in agitated behavior. Carefully selected music, based on that person's past preferences, can aid in stimulating remote memory—which remains intact longer than recent memory—and allow happy emotions to override the current stressors in the environment.

MUSIC AND MEMORY has been successfully employed in training family caregivers and also staff in long-term care homes. Using individualized music, specific to a person's prior likings, can help reduce distress. Research has shown that the program reduces anxious behaviors and the use of risky medications, such as antipsychotics, in people with dementia.

A fascinating documentary about this innovative program is *Alive Inside: A Story of Music and Memory.*

4. Touch is an important component in communicating with persons with advanced dementia.

Marcy and her mother often held Dr. Cottrell's hand and gave him frequent hugs. Even if they cannot tell you so, persons with dementia appreciate signals of affection through touch. Hold your family member's hand, let them know you love them, kiss them on the forehead. Touch is a method of communication that can reach deep without having to use any words. Soft items they can touch, such as a soft sweater or blanket, are also very soothing to someone with dementia.

5. Just being present with your loved one can be a form of communication.

When any sort of conversation is impossible, sitting quietly with your loved one is a powerful kind of communication: you are saying that they matter. The time you take to just be there is a message of utmost value, with or without words. You are providing a salient landmark in their ever shifting world.

6. Most of all, no matter how advanced their dementia has become, always treat your family member with respect.

This is communication at the most basic and most important level. Look your loved one in the eye, smile, and use a calm voice—even if they spilled ice cream all over the shirt you just spent 20 minutes getting on them! Always use gentle touch in everything you do and continue to show them you love them.

7. On a "bad day," when your loved one doesn't recognize you and doesn't want you to come anywhere near them, don't despair.

Dementia is a stressful disease in so many ways—for those who have it, maintaining their best cognition can be overwhelming and extremely tiring. When the disease is in the advanced stage, persons who have dementia are trying to make sense of a fragmented world and are often stressed by stimulation that family and caregivers don't understand (because there is no logic to it). Trying to make sense of worsening behaviors is frustrating and often futile. Rather, step aside and remind yourself that you are doing your best to partner well with your loved one, and offer some distraction (a bowl of ice cream often works wonders) and try again later.

Communicating with people who are deeply forgetful is not an easy task. It is, though, an essential one. Understanding that you are providing them dignity, offering them comfort and safety and ways to connect, is one of the most loving things you can do.

Clearly, though Dr. Cottrell had advanced dementia, he had moments when he could communicate his love for Margaret. Her gentle love every day continued to sustain him, and was what allowed him to find his "good days."

• 15 •

Do No Harm

There were clues something was wrong long before I stopped to think about it. Not knowing what to look for, I missed the emerging symptoms one after another. It wasn't until one hit me squarely between the eyes that I paused to look a little deeper.

Déjà vu. Four months after my father had been admitted to his new room, I discovered him lying in bed, unbathed, not dressed, unshaven, and with remnants of lunch on his sheets. I tracked down the first nurse I could find.

"He's like that because all the aides are afraid of him," she said, bluntly.

"Afraid? Afraid of what?"

"Your father's violent."

Never in a thousand years would I have dreamed such a gentle person could be described as "violent." Even at his worst with Alzheimer's, my father might have a sudden vocal outburst but then always quickly settled down.

"I don't understand," I said, confounded.

"He tries to hit them," said the nurse.

"Hit them!"

"He tried to hit me too, this week. To be honest, no one wants to change your dad's diapers or dress him anymore. He takes a swing at us when we put him in his wheelchair. He's always yelling something at us."

It had been several days since I had seen him, but this was news indeed. "He's never been like this before."

"That's because it's advancing," the nurse said knowingly. "Patients with dementia often get like this in the later stages. They can become real combative.

"I know it's hard to accept," she added, staring at my quizzical face. "Don't worry. I'll make a special point to get him bathed and shaved and changed today. I'll gather a couple of aides to help hold him down."

Returning to my father's room, I slumped in the chair next to his bed. He was sleeping deeply. I noticed the dirt under his fingernails and saw that his feet were tightly bound in the bed linens. I rearranged them. He didn't wake up.

Two days later my father was still not shaven, although he was up, sitting in his wheelchair. Instead of being in the Activities Room, however, where they often placed him during the day so that he could look out the window, he was in his room with the door closed. Reflecting further, I realized that for the past few weeks when I'd visited, he was always shut off in his room.

The aide had an explanation for this when I questioned her as she came to pick up his meal tray.

"He just won't take no for an answer," she said, turning to face my father and addressing him like a naughty two-year-old. "How many times do I have to tell you that you can't go into everybody else's room, George? And then you insist on going into our room where we hide the candy, scrounging through the drawers!"

"You hide candy?" I asked.

"Oh, it's just the little storage room where there's a desk. We often bring in cake or chocolates if it's somebody's birthday and keep it in there. Your father knows that, don't you, George?"

"So . . . what's so bad about that?"

"We can't have him going into the other rooms, you understand. And when we remind him, he refuses to move out. He acts like he thinks these rooms are his."

Perhaps he imagined them as his different examining rooms in his old office where he used to see patients, I mused.

"When we go to pull him out, he gets angry. And then he tries to go right back in! We must have told him a hundred times and he still doesn't listen!"

"That's why you're keeping him shut in here . . . in his room?"

"We don't have time to keep after him, you understand. The staff has tried locking his chair wheels, but somehow that doesn't seem to stop him."

The nurse smiled momentarily, "I don't think his poking around for candy is all that harmful," she added. "Lots of the elderly like sweets. But a bigger problem is George can't stand to be washed or transferred to the bathroom. He gets feisty—really mean to the aides. Lately, we've had to call in Fred—you've probably seen him around. Fred's hefty. He just scoops George up and dumps him on the toilet."

The nurse made a large swooping motion with her arms. "George screams and fights the whole time. All Fred's doing is trying to help."

After she left, I contemplated her words. It was a conundrum. If he insisted on roving, what else were the aides to do but restrict him to his room?

This was not the Alzheimer's unit where people mostly lived communally. Staring Susan, I knew, wouldn't do well in this nursing home section, either. With a whole new round of centrifugal emotions, I left Montavilla Prison in a vertigo of discouragement.

The following week I visited again, bringing my mother. We went straight to my father's room, but he was not there.

"He must be out and about," I said, relieved to find him not trapped in his room. His wheelchair was gone, too. "I'll bet he's in the lounge, enjoying the sights from the window."

But he was not in the lounge. My mother and I found him in the row among the Land of the Pink Bibs. He was situated near the end of the line, with the signature pink garment clasped around his neck. His head was bent down toward his lap, and though his eyes were open, they were not focused on anything. His shoulders slouched over, like a rag doll, and his mouth hung slightly open.

"Oh, not a stroke," said the nurse, when my mother asked her with alarm. She was not prepared for seeing him like this—completely subdued, saliva running from the corner of his mouth, resembling many of the other inhabitants. "He is fine," the nurse added, brightly. "He's just on a new drug."

"What's that?" I asked, suspiciously.

"Depakene. Doctor put him on it when we called him. George was getting bad—really bad. He was becoming violent to the girls. It's a mood-stabilizer."

"He looks drugged," I said.

"Yes, you're right. He is," she replied. "As you can see, he's really nice now. Controllable."

The nurse walked with us closer to my father and patted his head. "Hi, George. Your family is here to see you!"

He didn't move.

"You ate a good lunch today," she continued, cheerfully. "And when the aides lifted you to the toilet, you didn't shout. You were a good boy, George, not to hit." She patted him again. My father slouched further, the pink bib dropping into his lap.

My mother was completely speechless. My father, his head hanging even lower, did not have the wherewithal to acknowledge her presence.

"Keep on being a real good boy, and you'll get your candy! Maybe even a chocolate bar!" The nurse smiled and moved on, addressing now and then another patient. Many shared the same blank expression as my father, like they'd all had lobotomies, I thought, with a twinge of terror. Were they all sedated on mood-stabilizing drugs?

We cut our visit short; I wanted to get my mother home.

As soon as I dropped her off, however, I pulled out my cell phone to leave a message for the doctor. Returning my call after a few hours, he explained there was not much he could do except prescribe the mood-calming drug. The nurses felt threatened. Whenever they transferred my father to the bathroom, or to or from his wheelchair, or even merely moving him to bathe or shave him, he would bellow and howl. When they wouldn't stop what they were doing, he would beat at the air, or at them.

Though I hated to admit it, perhaps the doctor was right. Perhaps it was the only option if my father were that difficult to manage. What else could they do—except use a highly sedating medication to reduce his antagonism? They couldn't communicate with him when they were attempting to help him when the only word he apparently could say was "Ouch."

"So you're giving up, Mom?" asked Emily.

"Alzheimer's is one thing; violence toward others is another."

"But Papa's not like that," Jennifer said, agreeing with Emily.

"He is now." I wished I could put my own head down now on the table and forget everything. "Just put me in a pink bib and prop me against the wall," I said, tiredly.

"Mar, did you happen to see the paper today?" asked John.

"You know I haven't looked at the paper for weeks."

"Well, I think you better read this," he said prophetically, handing me an article.

"I would like to leave a message for Dr. Montgomery," I replied to an answering machine at the Florida State University Medical School.

I knew it was a complete long shot. After spending half a day trying to get the physician's number, I found it somehow and was actually routed by a receptionist to his voice mail.

"I recently read an article that you wrote about pain in the Alzheimer's patient—about how they can't communicate if they are feeling it," I continued, not knowing how much information to leave, yet suspecting this was probably my only chance to get his attention. "You see, my father was a surgeon in Portland, Oregon. He now has Alzheimer's disease and is in a nursing home. The staff there are saying he is combative and have sedated him. But after reading your research, I wonder, could he really be in pain and just not able to tell us?"

I highly doubted this busy, esteemed researcher—clear across the country from me—would ever return my call. Yet the story John had given me last night was riveting.

Dr. Montgomery was a geriatrician—a doctor of old people—and some of his research involved looking at severely demented patients who were experiencing pain but unable to express it in words. The article explained that a person suffering from Alzheimer's cannot reply to a healthcare provider who asks, "On a scale from one to ten—one being no pain and ten the worst pain possible—how would you rank your pain?"

Dr. Montgomery wrote that often the only way these patients can articulate their feelings is by yelling or flailing—out of fear and pain.

The article also said to be aware what medications were being administered to the patient. As I had not checked for a while, I called the nurse. As always, she sounded exasperated when talking to me. In rapid-fire recounting, she rattled through the list. I noticed that the Tylenol my father had been on initially for his broken hip was not on it.

"Oh, that hip shouldn't be bothering him anymore," she responded. "That happened many months ago. We DC'd the Tylenol. The rest of the drugs are just the same. The only new one is the Depakene. And that's been very effective."

Yes; it certainly was. It had "effectively" reduced what remained of my father's personality to little better than a worm, but worms had more energy.

The phone rang that night at dinnertime, and I was expecting it. I knew my mother had been visiting my dad that afternoon and that I would be getting another depressing report. I almost didn't pick it up but realized I was being cowardly. Emily grabbed it first. But the call was not from my mother.

"It's for you," said Emily. "It's Dr. Montgomery."

And so began a discussion with a man I had never met but who, in one long-distance phone call, changed all our lives. At nearly eleven o'clock for him, he listened to the entire story without interrupting, except for one or two questions. He acknowledged that what we were seeing was indeed distressing but unfortunately terribly common among patients with Alzheimer's disease.

"People like your father cannot elucidate their pain," he explained. "So we must be the detectives and figure it out. Did your father suffer from arthritis?"

"Come to think of it, yes. He often complained of back pain," I replied, remembering. "He had some shoulder pain too, like a nerve entrapment or bursitis, I think. And he had something called peripheral neuropathy in his legs, which made it difficult for him at times to walk."

"Your father is in pain," said the physician, unequivocally. "Do you know what medications is he on?"

I ran through them nearly as quickly as the nurse had this afternoon but added, "Nothing for pain. They said he didn't need it anymore."

"Well, they are very wrong. He needs something very much. Has he seen his doctor recently?"

"His doctor doesn't come to the nursing home. He said my father didn't need to be seen but should be put on the mood-stabilizing drug."

Dr. Montgomery cleared his throat. He sounded like he was going to say something but changed his mind. Rather, his tone took on a professional manner.

"I am very sorry about your father, Dr. Cottrell. You need to do three things right away. Do you have a pen to write them down?"

I grabbed a pencil and pad of paper.

"First, put your father on a regime of 1,000 milligrams of Tylenol, three times a day. That should dramatically reduce any combativeness.

"Second, make sure your doctor discontinues the Depakene at once. What your father requires is not sedation but behavior therapy, which means there needs to be better training for the nurses and aides on how to deal with patients with Alzheimer's. Your father is afraid of what they are trying to do with him and he can't understand what they are saying. Plus, they are causing him actual pain when they transfer him. That's a frightening place to be.

"Third, get a new doctor. You need a geriatrician who is familiar with Alzheimer's and will actually visit the nursing home to see patients. I know a good physician in Portland, Dr. Michael Hobbs. Tell him you talked to me and that I referred you."

Following the list of recommendations by Dr. Montgomery had immediate ramifications. The Depakene was stopped, Tylenol begun, and doctor changed. My father suddenly quit hitting. He stopped yelling when being bathed or moved in and out of bed. As his pain level diminished, his behavior significantly improved.

In addition to making drug modifications, his new physician, Dr. Hobbs, instructed the Montavilla aides to respond to my dad in a new fashion. He taught them about the powerful tool of *distraction*—instructing them not to yank my father out of a room, or handle him roughly, or confront him straight on. Instead, he told them, think of how you might parent a toddler who wants to do something you don't want him to. Rather than demanding compliance and staging a battleground, it's far more effective to sidetrack a behavior you don't want. To manage a frightened Alzheimer's patient, the better way is to use kindness and calmness. Never employ force, but draw heavily on diversion. Speak softly. Move slowly. Always act in gentleness.

Dr. Hobbs did something more. He saw to it that my dad got his sweets. He relayed to me that one day when he was visiting Montavilla he found my dad back in the storage room. A nurse was reproaching my father for rifling through the candy drawer and trying to scoot out of his wheelchair.

"I told her to stop scolding and to leave him alone," he recounted. "It wasn't a big deal, he wasn't going to eat very much, and it brought him some happiness. Plus, I explained that Dr. Cottrell was smarter than she realized. Every doctor knows chocolate is good for you."

With relief and gratitude, we watched my father transform from limp and unresponsive—glued to the wall or shut in his room—to smiling again, holding his head erect, and moving about. His life had changed—all because a pair of physicians looked at him not as a severely demented old man on a fast track to die but as a *human being*.

There are heroes in battle. There are heroes in peacekeeping. There are also heroes in medicine—those who practice the ancient oath to do no harm, to ease the suffering of our fellow men.

Our family knew two such heroes: *Doctors Montgomery and Hobbs*.

What I Wish I'd Known

The Problem of Pain in Dementia and Why Millions of Seniors Are Suffering

Elizabeth Eckstrom, MD, MPH, MACP

$\mathcal{A}$s Marcy and her family experienced, people with dementia are often no longer able to recognize that they are having pain, nor can they communicate to others that they are in pain. This presents one of the most serious problems facing older people and is too often undiagnosed. Rather than being able to express their pain, patients with dementia can only perceive that they are distressed. This can lead them to exhibit uncharacteristic behaviors—such as hitting, biting, rapid breathing, anxiety, and refusal to bathe or be helped onto the toilet. Reducing the suffering from pain is one of the most important tasks that family members and healthcare workers can do. Yet because it is not a straightforward presentation and is often unrecognized for what it is, preventing pain in a person with dementia requires several proactive steps:

1. While they are still healthy, talk with your parents to understand whether and what kind of pain they may have. Many older adults experience pain from arthritis, bursitis (inflammation of a bursa, the protective fluid in the joint), headaches, nerve damage, and a host of other reasons. This can be a challenge, though, as many older adults are hesitant to complain about pain, so their doctor (and you!) may not know about it or realize how much it bothers them. Also, find out what medications work for them to manage their pain. Document this for later so that you are prepared to help them if they ever need your assistance.

2. If your parent has dementia, make a checklist of prior pain problems, and frequently talk with your parent or staff at their facility about it. For example, if your dad has always complained of back pain but now doesn't, remember to regularly ask him if he has pain. *Play detective.* Watch your dad when he stands up or tries to lift something; see whether he grimaces or otherwise looks uncomfortable. Make sure that the staff at his facility are on the lookout for evidence of pain, too.

3. If your parent's behavior changes, don't forget to think about *new* sources of pain. Sometimes something as simple as an ill-fitting denture or a mouth ulcer may cause a person with dementia to stop eating, begin spitting out his food, or even start hitting his caregiver who is trying to help him eat. If any of these symptoms are observed, it is a clue that your parent needs to have a mouth exam to see whether there is a sore or other problem. Similarly, older adults with dementia may develop pain from an ear infection, constipation, an overly full bladder, or a urinary tract infection, as well as other types of infections or problems. Anytime a person with dementia starts exhibiting distressing behaviors, it is imperative he or she have a thorough exam to make certain none of these problems are present.

4. If a person with dementia begins to display troublesome behaviors and no obvious source of pain can be found, don't stop your investigation. Think back: did your parent have pain before developing dementia? Whenever uncharacteristic actions arise, it is always worth a trial of pain medications to see whether it may help your loved one. Pain treatment regimens are different, though, for people suffering dementia. While people of normal mental functioning are generally given pain medications "PRN," meaning "as needed," this doesn't work for those with dementia. Since they don't recognize pain for what it is and cannot express to anyone what they are feeling, they don't know how to ask for pain medication. It is imperative, therefore, that their pain medications be *scheduled*. In other words, pain relievers for those with dementia need to be given *routinely*, whether patients ask for them or not.

5. Over-the-counter acetaminophen (or Tylenol) is the best pain medication to try first, given at a dose of five hundred to one thousand milligrams three times daily. This is exactly what Dr. Montgomery suggested for Dr. Cottrell. At this prescribed amount, acetaminophen has the lowest risk of side effects of any painkiller and works very well for many types of pain. If acetaminophen isn't strong enough, however, there are alternatives to try, such as nerve medication and opiates, among others. All of these drugs, though, carry much higher risks of side effects and should be used only with very careful monitoring.

6. If your parent is suffering from pain, there is one more thing to remember: it is extremely important to utilize *non-medication methods* to help manage pain levels. Sometimes these will be enough to cure your parent's pain entirely. Several techniques have been shown to lessen pain and should be implemented with any pain treatment:

- *Daily exercise.* Walking, gentle stretching, and strengthening exercises all help in managing pain. Most care facilities and senior centers have excellent activities programs that older adults can benefit from.
- *Hot water bottles or heating pads.* Apply these on sore areas. Use caution, though, to prevent burns, for persons with dementia won't remember to turn off a heating pad.
- *Gentle massage and attention to positioning.* Both of these simple techniques can be incredibly helpful. Often they are overlooked. Older people who have pain should *not* spend too much time sitting in a chair or lying in bed. Lack of movement makes their joints stiffen and increases their pain. Older individuals need frequent movement and activity throughout the day to keep their joints lubricated. Repositioning also prevents sores from developing. "Move it or lose it" is only half the story. The other half is after it's lost, pain moves in.

Of all the suffering that goes with dementia, pain is one that all too often is unrecognized and ignored. Yet pain is one of the most common reasons people with dementia become distressed. It is often the primary reason patients begin exhibiting uncharacteristic and disturbing behaviors. With understanding of the problem, careful attention to the possibility of pain, and judicious use of the safest possible pain medications, this type of misery can be greatly reduced. Often the results of treatment of pain can be just as positive and successful as those Dr. Cottrell experienced.

· *16* ·

Return of the Man

$\mathcal{O}$n April 6, 2000, ten months after breaking his hip, my father died. He succumbed to viral pneumonia after being sick for only four days. Dr. Hobbs—who had become a trusted physician and advocate—walked with us through the last steps, helping us understand that what we were seeing was the final stage of Alzheimer's disease. His compassionate care allowed us to loosen our tightly held grips and not go to extreme measures, which would only terrify my father, and gave us the ability to let go.

We were all with my father when he died, surrounding him with love. Even the priest—who often came to Montavilla and had always tenderly welcomed my dad to the chapel—was there. My father knew his family . . . reached out to us . . . and there is absolutely no doubt in my mind that he recognized my mother. His last look of love was for her, alone.

A funny thing happens when a person with Alzheimer's dies, I came to discover. In your time of grieving, your *own* recent memory begins to fail.

For me, at first it happened bit by bit. A little fracture here, a larger one there. A peculiar sloughing started to occur, a breaking down of the shell that had built up and concealed the person I used to know and love. This breach in the encasement suddenly let in one ray of light, then another and another, until I began to see something I thought was lost forever: the real person that had been hidden just inside the barricade of Alzheimer's.

After my father's death, letters began streaming in. They came from people whose lives my father had touched. Many we knew, but there were also many we did not. We began receiving letters from patients, nurses, doctors . . . as well as the dean of the medical school, a university president, and the Academy of Orthopedic Surgeons. Strangely, they were not what I had been expecting after living for the past several years in the Alzheimer's universe. These letters communicated their condolences for the loss not of a demented, frail man who lived only a demented, frail life—but rather of someone we had nearly forgotten: my father, the man.

"Dr. Cottrell helped me and my mother, who was in the middle of a divorce and I'm sure tight financially, at a tough time in our lives when, without a father (mine died in 1947) I needed Dr. Cottrell's skill and reassurance. He was a great man. I'm sure he meant the same to the many he touched."

"Dr. Cottrell was a respected physician, teacher, and alumnus at Oregon Health Sciences University. . . . His colleagues and friends will remember him for his dedication and deep commitment to the practice of medicine."

"Dr. Cottrell was a remarkable individual whose life was one of distinguished service, genuine interest in other people, and great personal integrity."

"Dr. Cottrell's contributions to furthering knowledge in the field of orthopedic medicine and improving the lives of disabled children were unequaled in Oregon."

And possibly my favorite—from a patient who long ago had been a part of the Crippled Children's Program my father had started at the medical school after returning from World War II:

"In 1949, I contracted polio, and my parents were referred to Dr. Cottrell through Easter Seals and/or the Shriners. They were told I probably would not walk again. Since I was only four years old, I don't remember many details.

"Over the next 8–10 years Dr. Cottrell performed several successful surgeries on my legs and arm. I was able to walk and continue to this day. If it had not been for Dr. Cottrell, I do not know what shape my life would have become. He was a dedicated doctor and a leader of his time. I am sure there are many other people who share my experience and respect for Dr. Cottrell. He was indeed a great man!"

I handled these letters like a treasure. I read them over and over again. I made copies of them and pasted them in my journal. Like so many families struggling with Alzheimer's, I had been guilty of getting so caught up in his present ailment that I had lost the ability to see the true nature of the person he was.

I began to understand that the last months and years of my father's life weren't the whole picture after all. They were just a few snapshots at the end of a long film portfolio. The sad portraits were vastly outnumbered by the albums and albums showcasing a rich and full life. What's more, the final images weren't even put on archival photo album paper. While the rest of the pictures became sharper, the recent ones soon started losing their resolution, and many faded altogether.

My mother and I and our entire family mourned the loss of my father for a long time. But in that, I discovered a truth about Alzheimer's disease that I could not comprehend before my father died. I came to realize that when one dies of Alzheimer's, death takes the person away but gives something back in its place.

It returns our loved one.

II

A GOOD ENDING

Five Blessings of a Happy Life
(from the ancient Chinese)

Health. *With good health, anything is possible.*
Wealth. *Sufficient resources allow for comfort and improvement.*
Love of Virtue. *Goodness enriches one's life and the world.*
Longevity. *A long life bestows years of pleasure and joy.*
A Good Ending. *A peaceful passing . . . the final key to a
   gratifying life.*

17

A Radical Prescription

$\mathcal{C}$aregiving takes a toll on a person's health.

So does grieving.

The year after my father died was a time of mourning for our family, especially for my mother. While I missed my father terribly, I could not fully comprehend the feelings my mother was experiencing—losing a spouse of sixty-one years. That was a different kind of bond—more like a direct link to a person, inextricably connected. Perhaps what made it worse was the same thing that had made it best: the deep and profound love my mother and father shared.

My parents, long before Alzheimer's had set in, used to joke that they never wanted to be separated by death, so they had a plan. When their allotted time on earth was nearing its end, they would take off in my father's little plane and fly off together into the sunset. When the gas ran out . . . well, that was it. Time's up. They'd be together.

It didn't work out that way, of course. Life and old age got in the way. But now, without my father, the void in my mother's life was palpable.

A well-meaning but misguided friend who was also a social worker put it this way. The more devoted a couple was to each other, the harder the loss.

"In my experience, when a couple has been married for a long time, and have been especially close, like yours were, when one of them dies the surviving spouse doesn't last a year."

It was advice I didn't need. Yet it gave me cause for reflection as well as determination that my mother would not become another statistic. However, I felt some concern that there might be some truth in it. In the months after my father's death, my mother's health—which for eighty-five years had been strong—began to fail. Her life's new focus, and subsequently mine, was a revolving door of doctors.

At least once a week, it seemed, my mother got up, got dressed, had breakfast, and took a trip to see a specialist. These varied between ophthalmologists, orthopedists, cardiologists, urologists, endocrinologists, and dermatologists, as well as her internist. She visited because there were problems emerging with her eyes, heart, bladder, bones, skin, and thyroid. There were also issues with her hearing and allergies. On top of it all, her vigor and positive attitude had diminished, as well as her sense of purpose.

It was now close to a year since my father died as we drove to yet another appointment—this time to the cardiologist. My mother's most recent diagnosis was "atrial fibrillation"—a common disorder in older people, where the rhythm of the beating heart goes awry. To keep blood clots from developing, she was put on a drug called Coumadin that worked as a blood thinner to help prevent strokes.

While my mother agreed she did not want a stroke and complied with the Coumadin therapy, it was not without its risks. In many regards, it was a dangerous drug. It made the threat of falling even more serious. One never wanted to have thinned blood and hit one's head while on Coumadin. A blow like that could cause a major hemorrhage. For these reasons, the dosage was carefully monitored by professionals and its levels in one's blood checked regularly. The scientific name for the drug was warfarin. Which was another name for d-CON.

"It's hard to believe that I'm on a drug that Daddy used to kill mice," my mother sighed. She had not lost her quick thinking. "I'm just falling apart."

"No you're not. You're doing great," I responded. But we both knew that wasn't true.

"I wonder what new pills I'll get today. Every time I see a doctor I seem to get a new one. How many am I on now?"

I hadn't tallied them up, but there were plenty. "About eleven . . . more or less. That's counting your eye drops and nose drops."

"What are all these pills for?"

Stopping to think, I had to admit I didn't really know.

"Do the doctors know?" she asked.

"I'm sure they do," I replied. At least, I certainly hoped they did.

"You've been to so many doctors with Daddy and me that you probably could be one right now."

I didn't want to confess that I was growing a little sick of doctors; they were consuming my life. Yet once at the cardiologist's office, seeing a waiting room full of ill and fragile people and observing once more how feeble my mother was becoming reminded me to be grateful there was such a thing as physicians. We checked in, and I brought over some magazines for my mother to read. She shook her head.

"Lately, my eyes are getting so bad that it's hard to read the little print," she said, squinting at the periodical and then changing her mind and taking one.

One of the most devastating diagnoses that she had recently received was from the ophthalmologist. After running a battery of tests, the specialist determined she suffered advancing macular degeneration in *both* eyes. Being a voracious reader throughout her life, this came as a crushing blow. On a side table by her chair at home, she now had stacks of large-print books from the library. But even those were becoming more difficult to decipher, to her dismay.

The nurse called for my mother, and we headed back to the examining room. Expending effort to keep her balance, my mother hung heavily on my arm and shuffled her feet like they were stuck to the floor. Even with the small bit of exertion, her breaths were laborious.

"Dr. Vaughn will be right with you but first we need to get your weight," the nurse said. My mother, struggling to climb on the scale, refused to release my arm. "You've got to let go of her. You won't fall; I promise I'll catch you," said the nurse as she fiddled with the knob. "I just need to get your weight since last time. Why, you've lost eighteen pounds."

This was not good news. My mother didn't have that to lose. Once off the platform, we followed the nurse to the room, where she directed my mother to sit on the examining table. The doctor didn't come in immediately, and my mother complained that sitting upright on the bed hurt her back, but she didn't want to recline. With nothing to look at, she thumbed through the only magazine in the room—a color pamphlet featuring Viking Cruises.

"Daddy always hated cruises," she commented. "That's why we only went once. He said they were filled with a lot of old people sitting in chairs with blankets spread across their laps and not doing anything."

That image, unfortunately, now fit my mother perfectly.

"Good morning, Mrs. Cottrell," said the doctor, moving vigorously into the room. Dr. Vaughn was a young man with short-cropped, blond hair and a friendly face. "So how are you feeling today?"

"Okay," said my mother, weakly.

The doctor took the stethoscope from around his neck and put it in his ears. He listened to my mother's heart and abdomen, then took her pulse and tapped around a bit.

"I know it must still be hard for you, missing your husband." My mother nodded. "It takes time," he said gently. Picking up her chart, he reviewed it quickly. He closed it, laying it on the table next to a computer.

"Mrs. Cottrell, there's something you need to know," he said, looking into her eyes.

"Oh, no—" She was alarmed.

"Right now you are weak and frail. You've also lost eighteen pounds. That's more weight than I'd like to see. But it's not because of your heart."

"It's not?" She looked more distressed.

"No, it's not."

"What is it, then?" she asked timorously.

(I knew exactly what she was thinking, for the same supposition had been crossing my mind. Cancer.)

"It's because, Mrs. Cottrell," said Dr. Vaughn, "you're not exercising."

Possibly any other diagnosis would have been less startling than the one he spoke. My mother appeared dumbfounded.

"From your labs and the tests we have recently run, you are in exceptional health, Mrs. Cottrell."

"I am?"

"Yes, you are. You have the blood and lab results of a teenager. You are weak and frail because you have *stopped moving*."

Dr. Vaughn waited for the words to sink in. "You have lost your confidence because of your worsening vision, and you are anxious over falling. And, of course, you are despondent over losing your husband."

He moved in closer. "You need to start moving again, Mrs. Cottrell. I'm going to give you a radical prescription," he said.

"Another pill?" she asked.

"Not a pill. *Exercise*."

My mother looked disappointed. It was not the prescription she wanted to hear. She hated to exercise.

Dr. Vaughn had obviously faced this before.

"Mrs. Cottrell; I think you want to be around to see your grandchildren grow up. And right now your body is still capable of that. But your future is up to you. It's your choice. Get a walker—"

"A walker!"

"Yes, a walker. Your eyesight is compromised, as you know. A walker could add a little more support. And I want you to go to a mall, which is climate controlled. And *walk*. Take your daughter with you. Or go with a friend. Walking can strengthen your legs, improve your balance, and, in general, just make you feel better! Further, it will really help your spirits."

My mother softly groaned.

"And I prescribe a water exercise class for you, too, if you have a place to do it. That is easy on your joints and can help your knees and overall fitness. And when you feel up to it, have your daughter take you for a walk outside. Smell the roses. Go to a park. Above all, *move*."

I thought again of all the little old ladies in running shoes that my father had prescribed. He would have liked Dr. Vaughn. Leaving the cardiologist's office, I noted that my mother was more erect. She had stopped dragging her feet and even dropped my arm.

"He says I have the lab results of a teenager!" she reflected, still a bit stunned. A smile crossed her lips, then quickly faded.

"I would have preferred a pill."

What I Wish I'd Known

The Best "Anti-aging" Pill of Them All

Elizabeth Eckstrom, MD, MPH, MACP

If I, as your doctor, could prescribe a drug for you that could help protect you from heart attacks, reduce blood pressure, curtail diabetes, obesity, cancer, strokes, insomnia, depression, and Alzheimer's disease, as well as increase your brain capacity, you might be excited but doubtful. "What are the side effects?" you might ask. I would reply, "There are no side effects with this prescription. It will also cut your risk of breast cancer in half and lower your risk of bowel cancer by 60 percent."

Most people would say, "Okay, I'll take it!" but add, "But, Dr. Eckstrom, such a drug doesn't exist."

That's where the misunderstanding lies. Because there is such a wonder pill. It already comes in generic form, requires no waiting in line at the pharmacy counter, and, by and large, is free.

It's called *exercise*.

As Andy Coghlan reported in the August 2012 *New Scientist* magazine, "From dementia and diabetes to high blood pressure—no pill protects us against ill health like exercise does." Eric Richter, a research scientist at the University of Copenhagen, Denmark, states that there is probably not a single organ in the body that is unaffected by exercise.

But how does it work? The exact mechanisms still aren't entirely clear, but research has shown several key factors that come about from being active. Being overweight is a known risk factor in many forms of cancer. Exercise helps keep body weight at a safe level and thereby can lower your risk of developing cancer. Activity also helps clear blood vessels so that they can work as they are meant to, by helping to destroy dangerous fats before they clog up the system. Fewer fat deposits in the body also help reduce the level of exposure to potentially harmful hormones and inflammatory particles that adhere to them.

Other scientists are finding clues to the protective nature of exercise. One fascinating function is that exercise plays a vital role in acting in the capacity of—who would have thought?—a garbage collector. DNA is a material present in nearly all living organisms and is the main constituent of chromosomes. It is the "genetic code" stored in our cells and determines everything from how we are built to how we are maintained. DNA replicates; that's why we keep on living. But sometimes some of our body's DNA can become mutated or damaged. These problematic cells can become cancer promoters. Research by Beth Levine of the University of Texas Medical Center suggests that exercise can help eliminate some of these unwanted bystanders. Exercise "turns on" cells that hunger after additional energy and can burn up (not recycle!) potentially dangerous, loitering debris, some of which might be precursors not only to certain cancers but also to neurodegeneration and dementias.

Exercise also affects the hippocampus region of your brain—the part that is crucial for memory. In short, it can improve your memory by increasing its capacity. Exercise can stimulate new neuron development in the hippocampus. As the brain ages, memory function is known to decrease. Exercise, however, can hold back decline by increasing the volume of your hippocampus. Scientist Art Kramer of the University of Illinois has determined that this increase can "make up for approximately two years of normal age-related decrease."

Researchers are discovering other benefits to exercise. Being active excites mechanisms that work to reduce surplus glucose (sugar) in our muscle and fat cells; this, in effect, can prevent diabetes or even help reverse certain forms of the chronic and sometimes devastating disease. It also aids in enlarging small blood vessels. These healthy, dilated little circulatory systems can be life-saving conduits in the face of an impending heart attack or stroke. Exercise also can reduce pain from arthritis as well as increase your bone density and help you sleep better—all powerhouses in terms of quality of life in aging.

So if this magic "pill" is so effective against numerous diseases, increases your life expectancy, helps make your brain alert, and keeps dementia at bay for extra years, *why aren't more people taking it?*

Because it isn't just a pill you swallow. It takes a little work on our part. Exercise takes time many of us don't think we have. Yet this "prescription"—even if it requires some effort—more that any other remedy can buy us years of good living when we're older.

Marcy's mom wasn't very happy with the recommendation from her doctor. Many people aren't. But, as I will explain, there are ways around this that can be effective as well as fun. In a future chapter I'll describe the ideal exercise program and approaches to get your reluctant parent to participate.

Who knows? Maybe you'll join in. Exercise is not just for seniors. The benefits of being active can nourish and protect all of us for a lifetime.

18

No Senior Left Inside

My mother, motivated by the urging of my family and the haranguing of Alonzo, took Dr. Vaughn's suggestions to heart. We bought her a walker that a friend, a physical therapist, had recommended, called a Nova. It was bright metallic blue, lightweight, and could collapse to fit easily in the car. My mother took to it readily because it looked snappy and sporty—not like the bulky hospital version my dad had. *That* walker was stodgy and industrial, with four aluminum legs like stiff posts and cut-out yellow tennis balls affixed to the feet so that it could slide . . . with difficulty. The Nova wasn't like that. It was shiny and had wheels. It also had brakes on the handles like a bicycle. All the contraption needed, John said, was a new moniker and a Nike swoosh to make it a runaway best seller among the active geriatric set.

As Dr. Vaughn predicted, when my mother began to move, her health started to improve. Slowly at first, and in incremental units, the change was evident within a few weeks. After several months, her progress resulted in fewer visits to the doctors. She felt better, she looked better, and her energy level compounded.

At the local club, my mother joined water exercises for seniors two times a week. She liked the class because no one was under sixty-five and the instructor made sure they never got their hair wet.

Once a week she went to the mall—more often to shop than to exercise, but her growing stamina allowed her to enjoy the outings more. At least once a month she also took a day trip to the beach with Inez and Alonzo. There, she liked to go out for clam chowder or crab and maneuvered her walker in and out of coastal artisan shops. Even more, she loved to go out to lunch with me on our traditional Wednesdays—which we still tried to keep up even after my father died. On those Wednesdays when we didn't have lunch, we would go to the park, to the place that my father loved to walk.

Resulting from getting out more, her outlook perked up. She regularly came over for dinner, enjoying immensely feeling a part of the girls' lives. She got excited hearing about Jennifer's eighth-grade graduation ceremonies coming up and learning about Emily's favorite high school classes. She attended their events—Emily's choir concerts, Jennifer's soccer tournaments, and even the county fair, where they showed their sheep in 4-H. While she would never be a farm girl, she liked coming to the farm to see the animals, especially if there were little lambs.

"If only George could see me now," said my mother in early spring, stepping out across our pasture to see some newborns. Over her dressy beige wool slacks she donned knee-high black barn boots that she had purchased at our local feed store. "He wouldn't believe it."

"Papa would be so proud," said Jennifer, holding her hand.

"Now all you need, Nana, are some Carhartt overalls," said Emily, enthusiastically.

"Coveralls? *Never!*" proclaimed my mother.

We couldn't help laughing for the image was ludicrous. In the fullest sense of the word, my mother was a "lady." In her era, ladies didn't wear coveralls.

I wore coveralls.

At the same time as she was becoming more engaged with life, she never forgot my father. I came to realize that the most important part of her weekly routine was to visit the cemetery, which she did without fail. She always took fresh, white, fragrant daylilies to place on my father's grave. Somehow she seemed to have a special communion with my father there that she had nowhere else.

These were sweet months of respite; for a while we were able to experience a period of renewal. Even my mother seemed to be able to face the loss of my father with less sorrow and more hope. Things seemed to be reaching a new equilibrium, and on the eve of the second anniversary of my father's death, when I came to the house to pick up my mother for a trip to the cemetery, she met me at the door, ready to go.

"Look at you!" I said, surprised. "You're an ad for *Runner's World Magazine!*"

My mother had on a cute, peppy jogging outfit that I had not seen before. She wore a bright pink Nike zippered top with black sides, matching black running pants, and gray and white Brooks athletic shoes.

"On my walk last week I went to Nordstrom and saw this on display. I thought it looked quite sporty and comfortable, so I bought it. I think Daddy would like it."

"You're ready to start jogging with me!" I said, admiringly.

"Oh no, I would never go jogging," she retracted, smiling. "I just want to look like I do."

The ABC'S of Exercise

Elizabeth Eckstrom, MD, MPH, MACP

$\mathcal{D}$r. Cottrell was well ahead of his time in understanding the health benefits of exercise. All those older women wearing walking or jogging shoes to Nordstrom probably increased their life expectancy and improved their function in very important ways. However, when an older person isn't already in the habit of exercising regularly, as Marcy's mom was not, being told to exercise can be daunting. It is one thing for the doctor to say "You should exercise" and totally another for you to actually start a well-balanced exercise program. Many people commence but then quit. Others try for a while and then lose motivation. Still others don't know how to embark on a program or what even what a good exercise regimen is.

Let's begin with the foundations of what creates a well-balanced exercise program. We will then focus on ways to get motivated and stay motivated as well as techniques to prevent injury and avoid problems when starting to exercise.

THE IDEAL EXERCISE PROGRAM FOR SENIORS

Four key components make up the very best exercise programs. I call these *the ABC'S of exercise*. They consist of **A**erobic exercise, **B**alance exercise, **C**ore and strength exercise, and **S**tretching or flexibility exercise. Each one is essential for maintaining and improving health, safety, and quality of life.

1. *Aerobic exercise.*

This is exercise where you move enough to get your muscles warmed up and working together hard enough to raise your heart rate.

Walking, running, biking, and swimming are all fantastic forms of aerobic exercise; they improve your heart and lung function and can help you live longer. Numerous studies have shown that people who walk one to two miles per day live at least one year longer than those who do not exercise. If you combine this with a healthful diet and refrain from smoking, it helps even more! For older people especially, walking one to two miles every day or biking on an exercise bike for thirty minutes or swimming for thirty minutes are all excellent ways to achieve aerobic exercise. The next question is: "How hard to I have to push myself for that half hour?" There are two ways to help determine the level appropriate for you.

One is a simple calculation. Calibrate your maximum heart rate and then walk, ride, or swim fast enough to get your heart rate there. An easy formula to determine your maximum heart rate is: $(220 - age) \times 0.7$. The answer gives you a number you can strive for as a moderate intensity aerobic goal. For example, if you are seventy years old, your calculation would be $220 - 70 = 150$, then $150 \times 0.7 = 105$. If you get to this heart rate (beats per minute) and are feeling good, you can certainly work gradually toward a higher level of fitness, with a slightly higher heart rate, but this moderate goal will provide you important longevity benefits.

Another good way is to determine your *perceived exertion*. If, on a scale of 1–10, with 2 being "This is pretty easy," and 10 being "I think I'm going to pass out!" try to achieve an exertion level between 6 and 8 in your aerobic activity. In this way, as you become more active and in shape, this level can move with you, increasing your fitness and condition.

2. Balance exercise.

Many people think that walking is great for balance, but unfortunately, that is not true. In fact, research shows that people who walk regularly do not have any reduced risk of falls compared to those who do not exercise. Rather, it is essential to complement your aerobic activity with specific exercises for balance to lessen your chance of falling. For people over seventy years of age, studies have proved that the best balance training is to practice tai chi. As already mentioned in the chapter on fall prevention, tai chi has many more benefits than just cutting your falls risk in half. It has also been documented to lower blood pressure and cholesterol, reduce pain in people who have arthritis and fibromyalgia, improve sleep, and even improve your memory. For those who suffer congestive heart failure, tai chi helps them walk farther and longer. From a geriatrician's perspective, it's something that everyone should be doing. To reap the most benefit, you should practice tai chi for one hour three times per week.

3. Core and strength exercise.

Maintaining your strength gets harder and harder as you get older. This is truly a "use it or lose it" phenomenon. If you don't specifically work to strengthen your muscles, they will gradually atrophy, or deteriorate. Eventually, this leads to trouble getting up from a chair without using your arms and difficulty in doing household tasks and gardening. Lifting weights, taking classes in gentle yoga, and using brightly colored resistance bands that you can get from a physical therapist or sports shop all can help you improve strength. The good news is if you have already had a decrease in strength, you *can* build it back up again! Even people in their nineties who exercise regularly show impressive gains in muscle strength and ability to recover their function. In addition, strength training has the added benefit of helping to preserve memory—a critical piece as you age. Strength and core exercises should be done for a minimum of thirty to sixty minutes, two days per week.

4. Stretching or flexibility exercise.

Flexibility is increasingly hard to maintain as you age. Yet staying supple is a vital component to preserving your independence. As your joints get older, they stiffen up. Your muscles become less flexible. It becomes easier to be injured. Before long, you start to have trouble with things like getting in and out of the car, turning your head to see behind you when you drive, and getting up in the morning without feeling stiff and painful. Stretching is therefore an essential part of a comprehensive exercise program. Because flexibility is something so easily lost as you age, you should strive to do some stretching exercises every day of the week—even if only for ten minutes. Yoga is great for flexibility, as is gentle stretching before or after aerobic exercise.

At this point, you may be thinking: This sounds great, Dr. Eckstrom, but how do I make time for all this exercise? Let's get *real*!

You're right. Carving out time for exercise is a major commitment. But it is also a fact that its myriad lifetime health benefits far outweigh any seeming time inconvenience. If you will spend an hour a day on exercise, you will likely achieve years of better health. Yet many people have difficulty figuring out how to fit all the "ABC'S" into a typical week. There are many ways to do it, but here's one example that works well for many of my patients:

1. Three days a week, walk or bike for thirty minutes. Also do gentle yoga for thirty minutes.

2. Three days a week, swim or do another form of aerobic exercise for thirty minutes. Then, practice tai chi for thirty to sixty minutes.
3. Take a day off! Enjoy how great you feel!

Many people reading this, of course, will remain skeptical. A number will want to give up before they even start. This is especially true if you have never been regularly active and are pretty sure you really *don't* like to exercise—like Marcy's mom. For those like Margaret, who have never had an exercise program, this advice might seem completely overwhelming. If that's the case for you or your parent, how do you begin?

HOW TO GET MOTIVATED AND STAY MOTIVATED

You can get yourself going by taking one of many approaches. One good way is to try out *one* thing you like to do or to embark on something you have done in the past and enjoyed. If you have a friend who exercises, ask whether you might join her. Another fun option is to plan a lunch date twice a week with a friend that includes a thirty-minute walk and a relaxing lunch together afterward. If tai chi sounds a little intriguing, take someone with you and try out a class. One of my patients takes tai chi with her granddaughter three days a week! However, if these techniques don't work for you or you find you don't like the form of exercise you selected, don't feel bad or give up. There are plenty of alternatives. A patient of mine who used to enjoy swimming thought that it might be a good aerobic choice for her. But when she got to the pool, she realized she was too frightened of falling to attempt getting in and out of the water without assistance. She switched her plan and decided do take a tai chi class at the gym instead. This resonated with her and she loves it. Another patient decided to take up bicycle riding in his seventies. It was something he always wanted to do, but he assumed he was too old and weak to do it. He worked up slowly, building his strength and taking consecutively longer bike rides. Before long, he made a personal goal: to ride eighty miles in eight hours on his eightieth birthday! And he succeeded! Still another patient, age ninety-one, worked out a different method. Her goal was to remain in her own home, but she was becoming weak. She opted to try the strength classes several times a week at her nearby senior center; now she can readily get up and down the stairs in her home and do her own laundry and vacuuming.

So if at first you don't succeed, just explore something else! Think of it as an adventure; there are many ways to realize a good program.

But now comes the hard part. The bald truth is it's easy to get discouraged initially because you *won't* feel the benefits of exercise immediately. You have to stick with a program for three to six months to really notice that it is (1) giving you more energy, (2) improving your pain, and (3) helping with sleep. During this time, it's easy to lose motivation. For this reason, if at all possible, be sure someone else is either exercising with you or is helping to encourage you so that you don't lose momentum and stop too soon. We all need an Alonzo to egg us on!

TECHNIQUES TO PREVENT INJURY

Remember to do a few things when embarking on any new exercise program. First, talk to your doctor to see whether there are any considerations you should be aware of. Then, be cognizant that if you start exercising too quickly, it is easy to suffer minor injuries. It's perfectly normal to have mild muscle soreness when you initiate a new walking or yoga program, but if you are *very* sore after exercise and can't move the next day, it means you did too much too soon and should back off a bit. I always recommend never exercising *past* a point where you can carry on a conversation comfortably with a friend or, if you are lifting weights or doing yoga, where you start to feel too sore or unbalanced. Also, be certain to find a class that is geared to *your fitness level* and one that increases the intensity of the program very gradually. You will notice I didn't say your *age level*. Why? That's because some eighty-year-olds are more fit than many forty- or fifty-year-olds. The important thing is to find the regimen that works for *you*. Listen to your own body. For example, if your yoga instructor tries to push you harder than you think is good, find a different yoga instructor. If you try a tai chi class but feel unsafe doing it, grab a chair. You can begin by just sitting in the chair and doing only the arm movements. Then, gradually, try standing next to the chair, using it to hang onto. After a couple of months you will be pleasantly surprised to find that you *will* be able to do the tai chi moves without the chair for support, and you will feel wonderful.

Some people feel uncomfortable gauging their own exercise ability. This is where exercise trainers who have special expertise in older people can really help. These professionals can assist you in developing a personalized program that will keep you safe while improving your heart, lungs, strength, and balance. Many older adults who work with trainers two times a week experience great results in increased fitness, flexibility, strength, and energy.

AND REMEMBER

Always keep in mind the most important thing of all when you're exercising: *have fun*! A good instructor, other class members who become your friends, participating with your family, and the opportunity to learn something new can all make exercise a very enjoyable part of your day. More than that, it can help you to feel better all around and stay independent and engaged for years longer. Yes, it will take work; yes, it will take time; but it can change your life—whether you're nine or ninety-nine. So take a breath, look to a better future, and begin.

19

I'm Not Cedaring; I'm Scissoring

"*I*t's Alonzo," said Emily, handing me the phone. "He says Nana has a headache."

Jennifer was reciting her poem for the upcoming speech contest, and Emily was working on a chemistry problem with John's help. It was another night of homework after a busy school day.

"Her head hurts very bad," said Alonzo to me. "What do you want me to do?"

"Did you try Tylenol?"

"Yes. No good."

"How long has she had the headache?" I asked. Emily was complaining to John that there was no possible answer to the question posed in the textbook. Jennifer was still reciting. We were all a bit distracted with thoughts of holidays approaching; although it was still early December, pressure was already building, and the presence of Christmas was unmistakable. In many Portland stores, yuletide decorations had been up since Halloween.

"You want to talk to her?" said Alonzo, anxiously. "She's watching basketball on TV. You know she loves the Trail Blazers."

My mother obviously was waiting to speak with me and took the phone. "Marcy? Is that you? I don't understand why they won't talk to me."

"Who?"

"The Trail Blazers."

I was about to laugh and make a quip when I realized she sounded serious. "What are you talking about?"

"I think—I think I'm not tracking so well."

She had all my attention now. "You have a headache?"

"The Blazers won't talk to me," she repeated, sounding upset. "Maybe they'll talk to you if you call them." Her words were slurring.

"Mom, I'll call you right back," I said, immediately getting off the phone and dialing the doctor. In less than five minutes he had returned my call and advised taking her to the ER for evaluation. She had been off Coumadin the past few weeks in preparation for some scheduled dental work. Without it to thin her blood, there was always the chance that she could form a clot.

John asked whether I wanted him to go with me to the hospital. I declined; I knew I wouldn't be long.

"Is Nana going to be okay?" asked Emily and Jennifer, concerned.

"I think so; we're just checking. If anything comes up, I'll call."

I could make the drive to the hospital in my sleep. It was the same hospital where my father had spent his career as a doctor; where my parents went when they got sick or had surgery; where I was born and where my children had been born. By the time I reached the ER, my mother's headache had mysteriously vanished. So had her nonsense about the Trail Blazers. I was thankful she was cognizant, if a little blurry in her responses to random questions the doctor asked.

"I think it's Wednesday," she replied to the doctor, "and as for the president, right now I can't remember his name. I recollect voting for him and then regretting it."

He chuckled. "I can agree with that answer," said the doctor. He went on to order blood work and a CT scan of her brain to check for clots or bleeding. Everything came back normal. After two more hours of observation, he said he thought she was well enough to go home. When I asked what he thought had happened, he responded with a term I had never heard before.

"I have suspicions she may have had a TIA."

"What's that?" I asked.

"*Transient ischemic attack*. Or mini-stroke. A patient with atrial fibrillation, like your mom, is at higher risk for a stroke. Her tests showed her blood is thicker than it should be because she has not been taking Coumadin. This can be problematic. Sometimes, when the blood is sluggish, little clots can break off from a wall of an artery and can potentially block a blood vessel. If the clot lodges in a tiny vessel in the brain, it can temporarily block off the blood supply, causing a 'mini-stroke.'"

"So you think she may have had a stroke?"

"Mini-stroke," he corrected. "While the symptoms you observed in your mother—headache, confusion, difficulty in thinking—are similar to those of a major stroke, in a TIA, they are usually temporary and reversible."

"Thank goodness; I don't want a stroke!" exclaimed my mother.

"Should we be worried?" I asked.

"By their nature, TIAs can be unpredictable. You never know what's coming next," explained the doctor. "They can be numerous or sporadic. One person may have several TIAs in a single day, while another may only experience one or two over a period of years. The main thing we want is to try to prevent a major stroke from happening."

My mother nodded with a worried expression. "Me, too."

The doctor restarted her Coumadin and sent her home with instructions to have her blood retested next week. He said he hoped this would be the extent of it.

"I never thought I would become fond of Coumadin," my mother said, getting ready for bed. "And one good thing came out of this."

"What's that?"

"I get to cancel my dental appointment."

Two days later Alonzo called with the same anxiety in his voice. "You need to talk to your mother. She just woke up from a nap."

I hoped she wasn't trying to call the Trail Blazers again. I could hear Alonzo fumbling to put the receiver in my mom's hand. When she spoke, her tone was weak. "Hello—" she floundered. "I'm not cedaring."

I was hearing things. "What did you say?"

"My head hurts. I'm not cedaring," she repeated. "I'm scissoring."

Alonzo grabbed back the phone, panting. "See?"

I told him to call 911 and get her to emergency immediately. I would meet them there as quickly as possible.

Jennifer stopped practicing the piano and was staring at me, alarmed. "What's wrong with Nana?"

"I don't know. Can you call Dad?"

When I arrived at the hospital, the ER doctors were already tending to my mother. Alonzo told me they had ordered a CT scan but said that it might not reveal what was currently going on, which they believed was something they were calling a "*stroke in progress.*" He was wringing his hands.

Recognizing me, my mother pointed to her head while wincing in great pain. She tried to say something, but her speech was garbled. A nurse came in to check her blood pressure and said it was very high, 180/80, and uncontrolled.

Distressed, I took one of my mother's hands, but with the other, she continued holding her head and groaning. She was talking, but her words were coming out all wrong, in a frightening form of gibberish.

"Aphasia," said the nurse.

I asked her what she meant.

"It's when there's been an injury to the language area of the brain. They lose the ability to speak correctly. The doctor will explain."

When he did come in, the doctor reiterated that "aphasia" was the term they used to describe when someone was speaking in nonsense words. It commonly occurred in stroke victims. He said my mother also had something wrong with the reflexes in her right foot called "clonus." Too, she had right-sided "foot drag." Together, these revealed she had a right-side lesion in her brain.

"Does your mother have a DNR?" he asked.

I didn't understand the term.

"Do not resuscitate," he explained. "It's vitally important for all older people to have written instructions for times like this. Without a DNR, should your mother go into cardiac arrest, she will be given CPR automatically."

"Is . . . is that bad?" I asked.

The doctor placed his hand above her chest. "If I were to give your mother CPR, I would undoubtedly break her frail sternum. Pain would be immense, and she would likely never recover."

"Is she having a heart attack?" I asked, feeling more and more out of control.

"No. Does your mother have an advanced directive? A POLST? Those are end-of-life instructions. Who is her power of attorney?"

"I think I am, but I don't know," I said, completely bewildered by all the terms. "I remember signing something at the attorney's office—"

"Would you know where that paper is?"

"No."

"This is something I'd advise you to look into."

He left the room after saying we would know more after the CT scan was run. Completely befuddled now, I realized I'd forgotten to ask something of great importance.

I didn't know much about strokes, but what I had read from billboards, there was a thing called a "three-hour window" during which time doctors needed to act to avert permanent disability from a stroke. I remembered the advertisements said doctors could administer a "clot-busting drug" that could save a patient's life. Running into the hall, I searched for the doctor; it was nearly three hours since she had awoken from her nap.

"Do you need something?" said a nurse.

I asked for the doctor but had already forgotten his name. I said my mother was having a stroke and pointed to her room. "It's been three hours and she needs the clot buster, and she hasn't even had her CT scan yet!"

The nurse regarded me calmly. "I'll send in someone. Radiology is backed up. There are patients before her."

"But the window!"

"I'm sure the doctor will be in shortly," she said, turning into another room.

"Maybe we take her to another hospital if they're so busy?" asked Alonzo.

My mother continued whimpering and touching her head. To hell with the "no cell phones allowed" rule in the ER. I needed to talk to a doctor.

I dialed the first one I could think of, a friend and trauma surgeon. Miraculously, he was home. He listened to my own form of aphasia as I frantically explained about my mother, asking him what to do. There were only minutes left to act . . . to try to save her life!

"I think the best thing you can do is let God take control now. The doctors are doing the right thing," said Tom.

"What do you mean? It's been three hours and she needs the clot buster!"

"That procedure could kill her," he countered. "You said your mom is eighty-seven and on Coumadin therapy. Doing an aggressive tPA could likely have the opposite results from what you want. It could produce a major brain bleed. Call me when they have the results of the CT scan. Let go and let God."

"Did he say move her?" said Alonzo, with one hand already on the rail, ready for action.

"No," I said. "We wait."

The CT results, when they were finally run, didn't show much of anything, only revealing it was still a stroke in progress. The doctor had my mother admitted to the hospital. She was still in severe pain. At nine o'clock that evening, John came with the girls, and I sent Alonzo home.

"Do you want me to stay? You can go home and get some rest," John offered.

"No, I want to be here tonight. I'll just curl up in this chair next to her and try to get some sleep. At least," I said, trying to smile, "it's not a conference room."

An hour after everyone had left, I closed my eyes. Taking her hand in mine, I tried to remain calm each time I heard her moan. I was just falling asleep in a twilight of uncomfortable, discordant dreams, when I felt a finger rapping my shoulder.

"You can't be in here," said the night nurse abruptly. "Sorry."

"What?"

"You'll have to leave now."

"But I want to be here. She's my mother!"

"It isn't allowed. If you're planning to stay all night, you'll have to sleep down the hall, through the double doors, in the area marked "waiting room.""

"But I want to be with her!" I repeated, dully.

She placed her hands on her hips, standing with authority. Right then I knew I'd lost the battle. The nurse waited until I got out of the chair and picked up my purse, making sure I wasn't going to fall back asleep.

With the same finger, she motioned to the right. "Through those doors. You'll find some couches there."

What I Wish I'd Known

How to Ensure Parents' Wishes for Care Are Met—*Before* a Crisis Hits

Elizabeth Eckstrom, MD, MPH, MACP

One of the hardest but most important things we all must do as we get older is to ensure that our children and/or close friends know what our end-of-life wishes are. But how is that done? And how can we make sure those desires are truly met?

This puzzle has several critical parts. The work you do at the outset to put them all together and in the order that best fits you will pay immeasurable dividends in the future to you and your family.

To guarantee your wishes are followed, you need to draw up a will and designate where your assets will go. You should choose someone to represent you if you can't make your own medical decisions, and beyond that, try your best to communicate what treatments you would want should something happen and you no longer can make your own care decisions. For most older people, all of these tasks are complicated, and for some, they may be downright loathsome. Additionally, many older people have several children and are uncomfortable having to choose one to represent them. On top of that, it is always easier to put off talking about end-of-life wishes or planning for a time when you are no longer able to care for yourself. Yet the time will come for all of us when these points become crucial to address. Therefore, if these decisions are contemplated, discussed, and enacted early, done together with everyone who matters, it will provide enormous relief to all.

Being a doctor, I am going to focus on the medical aspects of planning for future healthcare decisions. These fall into three general categories, many coming with a confusing array of acronyms: (1) naming a power of attorney, (2) completing an "advance directives" form, and (3) formulating a physician order for life-sustaining treatment. I will discuss each in detail, for they all play a role in making certain your wishes are explicitly set forth.

POWER OF ATTORNEY FOR HEALTHCARE (POA OR POAHC)

A *power of attorney* is a person, selected by you, who will be the one to make decisions if you have a medical problem that renders you incapacitated to decide things on your own. For example, if you develop a temporary disease (e.g., a heart attack or infection) that alters your thinking or have a more gradual disease (like dementia or schizophrenia) that makes you unable to think clearly, a POA will represent you and make certain your wishes are followed. Marcy's father had Alzheimer's dementia, and eventually his mental status was poor enough that he couldn't make decisions for himself anymore. Marcy and her mother had to make health determinations for him. In some of the situations, they didn't have conversations before his dementia to know exactly how to best follow his wishes (such as choosing a facility) and so had to make their best guess. This can be hard for family members.

Other issues can emerge if there are many family members involved, each with differing health beliefs. It is therefore important to choose a POA whose health viewpoints are most consistent with your own. After that selection is made, plan to get the rest of the family members on board to allow the designated POA to be the decision maker. It is wise to also designate an alternate POA in case the POA isn't available when needed. And this doesn't mean that no other family members can be involved—hopefully, these early discussions will ensure that the entire family can come to agreement and support the POA in making decisions in a time of crisis.

In some situations where family members are not in agreement, this can be easier said than done. Often it requires multiple conversations among the entire family, which can be problematic if some family members haven't spoken to each other for twenty years. But before the need comes up is the time to get the communication channels opened again. When things are not left in order and wishes clearly delineated, unfortunate circumstances can occur. Many times I have observed an estranged son or daughter rushing in at the last moment to try to get a breathing tube put down Dad. These unfortunate situations have disastrous consequences for everyone involved.

ADVANCE DIRECTIVES

Advance directives are written instructions, set forth by you, stating how you wish your medical treatment to proceed if you are unable to make the determinations for yourself. Every state is different, but most allow patients to leave written instructions that their power of attorney can follow if necessary. There are three major provisions that you need to think about when completing advance directives, all of which can be a little confusing. For this reason, I address them separately: cardiopulmonary resuscitation (CPR), mechanical ventilation (utilizing a breathing tube), and artificial nutrition.

CPR or Cardiopulmonary Resuscitation

If you were found without a pulse (your heart had stopped beating) and without any respirations (lungs had stopped working), would you want someone to push on your chest, likely breaking your ribs or sternum, shock you, put a breathing tube down you, and try to bring you back? This question is best answered by asking a second question: *What are my chances of coming back to be who I was before if someone did this to me?*

The answer is relative to your age. If you are in your twenties and have a car accident and someone finds you within a few minutes, you could have a full recovery after cardiopulmonary resuscitation, or CPR. However, if you are over seventy and have CPR in the hospital, your chances of surviving it and living to be discharged from the hospital are only 2–17 percent. Worse, studies have proved there is a high probability that survivors will have a greatly reduced quality of life and regret having had CPR. For those having CPR performed in nursing homes, the record is even more sobering, with one large survey showing no one surviving. Other research has documented that elderly persons found without a pulse or respirations outside the hospital or nursing home setting have practically no chance of meaningful survival.

Since the outcomes are dismal at best, many older people find choosing *not* to have CPR a straightforward decision. This involves specifying a DNR (do not resuscitate) order. With such a low chance of survival, most people do not want to go through all the harsh procedures, but the choice, of course, is yours.

Mechanical Ventilation (Utilization of a Breathing Tube to Stay Alive)

Sometimes persons will have respiratory failure—they stop breathing—while their heart is still pumping. In these instances, you would not need chest pumping, and a breathing tube could save your life. However, if you have a serious lung disease, such as emphysema, and need a breathing tube to survive a respiratory failure event, there is a real possibility that you will never be able to breathe on your own again. Therefore, it is important to discuss your health condition with your doctor when deciding to choose (or not to choose) a breathing tube if there is a good chance you will never be able to breathe without it again.

Artificial Nutrition

If you come to a point where you cannot eat or drink on your own, artificial nutrition becomes necessary to keep you alive. To provide it, a tube is put into your stomach to give you essential liquid food and water. For some people, after enduring a major stroke or severe illness, it is entirely possible to have a feeding tube inserted for a few days or weeks to get through an acute problem and then subsequently recover. However, it is important to clarify in your advance directives whether you would want a feeding tube under conditions where there was little or no chance that you could *ever* eat on your own again or continue to live without tube feeding.

Completing your *advance directives* is an important tool to assist your power of attorney in knowing what you would want in the case of an emergency. It has one serious limitation, however: it doesn't guarantee that the paramedics who come when 911 is called will follow those wishes. For this reason, some states (Oregon was the first) have developed an additional form to ensure that your wishes are enacted:

PHYSICIAN ORDER FOR LIFE-SUSTAINING TREATMENT (POLST)

POLSTs, or *"physician order for life-sustaining treatment"* are forms that help elucidate your wishes to paramedics and emergency teams. After discussion with you, they are filled out by medical doctors, nurse practitioners, or physician assistants to translate what you want into orders that paramedics and emergency teams must follow. It is important to complete this form with the primary care clinician who knows you the best and thereby be sure he or she is representing your exact wishes.

Marcy learned about the POLST the hard way—in a crisis situation. This is the absolute worst time to have to think about such difficult questions! When someone is in the midst of an emergency, it is hard for anyone to think straight—even the medical professionals who at that point are simply trying their best to keep your loved one alive. POLSTs, therefore, can provide imperative information when urgent decisions have to be quickly made.

For more information about the POLST program and to learn whether it is something you might like to do and whether it is available in your state, please see polst.org.

As a geriatrician who regularly deals with these situations, I am fully aware that all of these conversations are difficult to bring up. No one wants to think about what might occur near the end of your life. For that reason, a majority of older adults and their families have not discussed them. But, as I have witnessed, the "head-in-the-sand approach" makes for the possibility of even worse outcomes and increased suffering for the entire family.

So how do you begin tackling such hard questions? In my experience, I have observed that it's best to have these conversations early, allowing all parties to express their views openly. Then, after listening to them and taking their views into consideration, come to an agreement and write down the results that best fit *you*. Next, select a power of attorney who shares your views so that if someone in the family does not agree, he or she will still need to accept what you have articulated as your wishes and not try to fight them. Your doctor and healthcare providers can help you and your family with these issues and aid you in coming to agreement about tough options. So be sure to include your primary care clinician in your conversations, especially if you are struggling to make decisions.

It takes time and courage to talk about these issues. But the bottom line is this: the work and thought you invest now—long before any emergencies arise—can be one of the most loving things you can do for those who mean the most to you.

• *20* •

Who's Shelby?

*W*hile I couldn't officially be in her room, that didn't mean I couldn't be in and out of it all night. Until her headache began abating, I didn't feel safe leaving her alone. And I didn't like all the talk about POLSTs—whatever they were. It seemed like everyone expected her to die. Moreover, the couches were short—more like love seats. There was no way I could sleep with my long legs dangling over the end. I considered sprawling out on the floor but was afraid someone might call security.

But I must have fallen asleep, for as dawn approached, a nurse with a gentle voice called me to wake up.

"Shelby? Your mother would like to see you."

Quickly glancing around the waiting room, I saw no other person. The nurse must have the wrong daughter. "I'm not Shelby."

"Is your mother Margaret in room 672?"

I nodded.

"Well, she is asking for you, Shelby. I'll take you back to her."

I was full of questions as I trotted alongside. "How is she this morning? How's her blood pressure, her headache?"

"Both are better," the nurse said, leading me to the room. "Here she is, Margaret. I found Shelby!"

My mother's face broke into such a sweet smile that I didn't care what she called me just then. I could be "Artichoke" for the rest of her life. All that mattered was that the twisted contortion of pain seemed gone from her face and there was a brightness to her eyes that I didn't know I would ever see again.

"Shelby!" said my mother, reaching out a frail arm attached to an IV drip, toward me.

133

"The neurosurgeon is already at the hospital, making morning rounds. He should be by to see your mother shortly," said the nurse. She checked my mother's blood pressure and pulse. "135 over 80; much better, Margaret. And I know you're happy Shelby's here."

"My Shelby—" said my mother again. She touched my hair lightly with her free hand. "I love you."

"Mom, how much I love you!"

She regarded my face, like she was trying to take it all in. I knew I looked a wreck. "Lorgeous," she said, squeezing my hand, gazing at me. "You are lorgeous."

"Lorgeous? I think you mean gorgeous? Oh, I look awful."

"You're lorgeous," she said again. Then she started to laugh, staring at the hall outside her door. "Uh-oh, Shelby; they shouldn't be doing that."

"Doing what?"

"Kissing."

I looked into the hallway. There was no one there but a nurse regarding a chart that she held in her hands.

"Don't you see them?" my mother asked. A naughty little smile crossed her lips. "They're supposed to be working. They shouldn't be kissing like that. Don't *stare* at them, Shelby."

My mother turned her glance toward the bathroom door, at a dirty laundry hamper. "My, what a pretty German shepherd," she said. In no way could I visualize the hanging bag into a German shepherd. "He's been here all night. He hasn't left my side."

When the neurologist arrived a half hour later, I realized I might need his help, too, for I was feeling more baffled by the minute by my mother's soliloquies. He said there was good news and bad news. My mother's CT scan revealed evidence of a previous small stroke, but the good news was she didn't appear to have any permanent disability from it. The bad news was she could have another TIA at any moment, or worse, a major stroke.

The doctor went on to say he wished to keep a close watch on her "stroke in progress" and also run an MRI and MRA to investigate the blood vessels in her neck and brain. He prescribed an increase to her Coumadin dosage and added a new drug, Plavix, to try to help ward off more clots.

"We will have a better idea what we're facing after these tests come back," he said.

"Shelby should have been a doctor," interjected my mother, proudly. "She would have been a good doctor."

The neurologist was jotting notes in his chart. "I'm sure she would have, Margaret." Putting down his pen, he took in my unkemptness. "I think she needs some rest. Go home, Shelby."

As one doctor called it, we were now on a roller coaster. "Put on your seat belt and get ready for the wild ride."

I never liked roller coasters. They frightened me and made me feel sick. Another physician said it's like your life is now attached to a yo-yo. The better term, I thought, was "boomerang"—for that was exactly what my mother seemed to be doing.

On Saturday, she improved. On Sunday, she had an "episode." She declined on Monday. On Tuesday, she improved again.

In all, she had five mini-strokes in seven days. Seat belts, I realized, weren't enough for this journey. We needed air bags.

The neurologist was equivocal in his prognosis. On the one hand, he said he was encouraged by her "lucid moments" between the TIA events. On the other, there was always the probability that she could go downhill and suffer a major stroke and permanent disability. He was less concerned about the hallucinations she exhibited during the "bad" moments.

"They're commonplace," he said, after my mother had just told him for the third time about the noble German shepherd dog that continued to lie protectively by her bed. She also asked why I was growing a beard. "Patients like your mother are often woken up throughout the night—for blood draws, IV infusions, blood pressure monitoring—so their sleep cycle is disrupted. In someone who is fragile, it can send them into more of a delusional state."

"Will she come out of it? Be like she was before?"

"Most likely she'll come out of it. But be just like she was before? At her age, that's always hard to say."

Test results were a combination of both good and bad. They showed no narrowing of the major arteries, such as the carotid—a positive sign—but revealed narrowing in a tiny artery in the cortical cortex part of her brain. This stubborn, problematic vessel was the site where each of the tiny clots got *stuck*, said the neurologist, and produced the aphasia episodes we were seeing.

"We call them "stutterings," said the doctor. "There's no surgery to cure this form of micro-vascular disease. The best therapy is the one she's on— blood thinners. And while they reduce the risk of a major stroke, they don't eliminate it.

"All life is unpredictable," he concluded. "But this is the most unpredictable you can get."

After he left, I sat with my mother, who fell back to sleep. I knew I hadn't slept well either this past week. And a frightening thing was, I was beginning to see the German shepherd dog too.

But something happened at noon. My mother *woke up*.

"Good morning, honey!" she said, with clarity and strength in her voice. Her eyes, too, were surprisingly clear. "I'm hungry!"

A gush of relief swept through me. "You're hungry?" She had not eaten much for over a week.

"Yes I am! I'm actually quite hungry."

I stood up and stepped around the sleeping dog. "Then I'll check on your lunch. They already took away your breakfast tray. I'll ask at the nervous station."

"Darling," she called after me, laughing, "I think you mean *nurses'* station."

After that, there were no more TIAs or stutterings. From that moment, she improved. She convalesced so rapidly, in fact, that the stroke nurses, the neurologist, and her internist were surprised. All her delusions stopped entirely. Shelby left. My beard was gone. Nurses ceased philandering in the halls. We started talking about Christmas. There was one thing I missed, though—the faithful German shepherd dog. It, too, had disappeared—possibly to help another sick patient.

With the aid of a physical therapist, she graduated from being in a wheelchair to learning to walk again. Four days after the termination of her TIAs, her foot drag was nearly unnoticeable, though her balance still needed work. Her overall strength was remarkably better as well as her outlook.

The best news was that the neurologist said she was recovering so well that she could go home.

Emily and Jennifer were overjoyed. "Let's have a party for Nana!" declared Jennifer. "We can make a 'Welcome Home' sign and have a Baskin Robbins ice cream cake. And we should also get a Christmas tree for her."

Alonzo was happy, too. He volunteered to make his specialty—a paella—which he produced anytime there was even the slightest reason to celebrate. Inez, of course, was invited. My mother, learning of the plan, thought it grand and said she couldn't wait to have real food and get out of a hospital gown.

"We'll leave the 'lorgeous' flowers here, for the nurses," she laughed. "Lorgeous" had become a new word in all our vocabularies. So had "Shelby." My mother never could figure that one out. "I've never liked the name Shelby," she said. "Where did that come from?"

The night before she was to be discharged, we left her in a cheerful mood. Several nurses came to say good-bye and wish her happy holidays. She had charmed them during the past week when she was more herself, and the attentive physical therapist who was so pleased with her progress had even begun calling her "Precious." Everyone agreed it had been a worrisome two weeks; I relished the idea of life getting back to normal.

"Shelby, dear," she kidded, "do you think we could stop by Starbucks for a mocha when you come to get me tomorrow morning?"

My mother loved her mochas. "Of course!" I replied.

But there were to be no mochas. The following morning, before ever reaching my mother's room, I was accosted in the corridor by Jan, a hospital social worker.

"I'm sorry, but your mother won't be going home today," she announced. "She'll need to go to a skilled nursing facility to recuperate after the accident last night."

The planets were rearranging in my mind. "Who—why—what are you saying?"

"After her fall."

"What fall?"

"Your mother fell in the bathroom last night."

"But nobody called me!"

"We all will know about her condition after the x-rays," she offered in a professional manner.

"X-rays? Did she hit her head?" I cried. "She's on blood thinners!"

"I said we'll know more after the x-rays," repeated Jan, coolly. Nearing her office, she turned, leaving me standing alone in the hallway.

What Is a TIA? And What Do I Do If I Think My Parent Is Having One?

ELIZABETH ECKSTROM, MD, MPH, MACP

$\mathscr{A}$ transient ischemic attack (TIA) is an interruption in brain function that results from a temporary deficiency in the brain's blood supply. It occurs when small pieces of fatty matter or calcium, adhering and built up on an arterial wall, break off and become lodged in the small blood vessels in the brain, momentarily cutting off blood supply. It can also happen when clumps of platelets or a blood clot block a blood vessel for a short time.

Symptoms of a TIA are scary. They look like someone is having a stroke. For example, someone having a TIA might have a droopy mouth and slurred speech. They may have difficulty in finding the appropriate words or saying them. They may experience imbalance, double vision, or weakness or paralysis of an arm or leg. Fortunately, most TIAs are just that, *transient*, and resolve quickly and completely. Many persons, after experiencing one, may be totally back to normal within twenty minutes. But while TIAs do not necessarily lead to lasting disability, they should never be ignored. They can be a harbinger of far worse things to come with more lasting effects—such as a major cerebrovascular accident or stroke.

If you witness a parent having what may be a TIA or a care facility calls to tell you your loved one has just had an "unusual event," it is vital that your parent be evaluated right away. If the primary care provider has the ability to see your loved one within a few hours, it could be possible to prevent a trip to the emergency department; if not, then seeking urgent care is essential.

Like Marcy, many people have heard about the "three-hour window" that is so crucial for treatment of a major stroke. This same window, however, does not apply to a TIA. Why? Because people experiencing a TIA do not need the same intensive therapies. Yet it is still critical to *assess* TIA patients to help determine their risk of developing a full-fledged stroke within the next few days or weeks. After having had a TIA, the probability of suffering a major stroke can be significant. Therefore, it is imperative to determine what further workup or medications might help reduce that chance. Because Marcy's mother had atrial fibrillation—a heart condition that can lead to the creation of small blood clots—she was put on a drug called Coumadin—a blood thinner, proved effective in reducing the risk of developing dangerous clots that can lead to more lasting events. Like many blood thinners, though, this drug needs to be closely monitored.

The treatment of all TIAs is for one thing: to prevent a major stroke. If you see symptoms, don't wait. Seek immediate evaluation. In other words, make sure to find help for your loved one before this "trial run" becomes a lasting event.

• *21* •

Stories from the Fall

I heard a terrible story once, told by a friend who had lost her father. He had been transferred to a local nursing home to recover from routine heart surgery. The following morning, she was called at 6:00 a.m.

"What do you want us to do with the body?" asked the attendant.

The "body" was her father, who had died overnight.

My mother was alive—barely—but no one could tell me what had happened to her. The story changed according to who told it. Jan said my mother had asked to be taken to the commode, and the nurse had "just stepped out to give her some privacy." Another nurse said that my mother had gotten up to walk to the bathroom in the middle of the night by herself and then tripped. She said my mother called for the nurse, who came immediately running. Yet another account was that a night nurse, after helping my mother to the toilet, left her, assuming she could get back in bed by herself.

Upon entering my mother's room, I found a different person. She lay in her bed with one hand putting her hearing aid in her mouth and the other pointing to the ceiling while mumbling nonsense songs. The motions, so reminiscent of my father in advanced Alzheimer's, were devastating to see.

"Oh, Mother; I am so, so sorry," I whispered, unable to hold back tears.

Taking the hearing aid from her mouth, I could only stare with overwhelming sadness. She began to pick and pick at her bed, her blanket, her hospital gown. Recoiling, I cringed; my God; not that repetitive picking! I tried putting her hearing aid back in her ear. Immediately, she pulled it out again, with a terrible vacancy to her gaze. She put it back in her mouth. Gently, I took it away.

Striding to the nurse's station, I asked when the x-rays would be done and was told at noon. There, I got a fourth recital—this one that an aide on the night shift had taken my mother to the bathroom and waited there with her. The aide had "turned her back only for an instant" when my mother tripped and fell. That did not quite agree with the story I heard from the occupational therapist an hour or two later. She said she'd heard that a nurse had been with my mother, holding her the entire time while she was on the toilet, only she lost her grip when my mother accidentally fell backward.

Adding them up, I counted five different scenarios. There was a funny thing about all of them, though. No one could tell me (1) who the nurse was or (2) what time the fall occurred. Before long, I began to suspect the obvious—no one really knew what had happened because no one had been with her. She had fallen to the floor sometime in the night and was discovered later.

Once back in the room, I made some calls and sat with my mother to wait for her to be taken for x-rays. She was obviously in pain but couldn't elucidate where. Her internist, Dr. Moore, ordered x-rays of her hip, back, and pelvis to look for possible fractures and also a CT scan to check for bleeding on the brain.

At twelve thirty, while we remained in the holding area for radiology, I stroked my mother's head. She was awake but highly confused.

"Mom, do you know who I am?" I asked.

She fixed her eyes on my face. "No."

"It's me. Marcy."

"How do you spell it?"

The question was so peculiar it took me by surprise. "M-A-R-C-Y."

"Oh, that's good. I never liked M-A-R-C-*I-E*. You are a nice nurse. But who is taking that shower?"

"What shower?" I asked, feeling sick.

"In the room right behind us. Don't you hear it?" She paused to listen and nodded like she assumed I heard it too. "I think it's George. He certainly is taking a long shower."

My mother reached up to remove her hearing aid and tried putting it back in her mouth. Again, I fished it out, dried it off, and replaced it in her ear. "Oh, Mom . . ."

She grimaced. "Can't you do something for my back? It hurts so much!" She started picking at the sheet. Not being able to stand it, I reached for her hand and put it in mine.

"I'm worried," she said, frowning.

She was worried? I was petrified. "What are you worried about?" I tried speaking calmly.

"I don't know what to get Mother!"

I gasped. "What did you say?"

She formed her words again very clearly. "I don't know what to get Mother for her birthday. It's coming up, you know."

When the radiologist came for her, I wilted back in the chair with my head in my hands. Then, I realized with a shot of panic, I should have taken the hearing aid out; she might be trying to eat it right now. Yet when they were through, which didn't take as long as I expected, it was still in place.

The aide took us back to the elevator and up to the room. Once situated, my mother asked to go to the bathroom. I rang for the nurse.

"I'll have to get some help; she is a two-person transport," said the aide.

It was difficult to comprehend that just last night my mother was anticipating going home; now all her advancement had evaporated. As the afternoon progressed, so did her pain. Dr. Moore, when he at last came by, was disappointed.

"What a shame; she didn't need this," he said, regretfully. "Thankfully, the x-rays show no hip, pelvis, or leg fractures. She has broken some lumbar vertebrae. The upper vertebra, L1, will be disabling for a while and cause her discomfort. She also suffered several broken ribs."

He concluded by reiterating what the social worker had said: my mother would not be going home. She needed further care at a skilled nursing facility.

"She is so mixed up," I said, feeling frantic. "Do you think her confusion is another stroke?"

Dr. Moore did not think so. He did not even call it a stroke in progress or TIA. He explained that such an "acute event," like this accident, could bring on confusion.

"I'm not leaving her alone again, here," I declared to John, who came by after work, bringing Emily and Jennifer. Alonzo was visiting too. "I don't care if they have a fit or not; and I'm not staying down the hall on the couch. Someone is going to be with my mom from now on."

"I will stay," offered Alonzo. "You need rest."

"Nana's crying, Mom," said Emily, looking frightened. "She's mumbling something."

We all stopped to listen. She was whimpering. Her words were pathetic: "Please help me!"

"What's wrong Nana!" exclaimed Emily.

"Please help me," she groaned, reaching for Emily's arm. "They won't help me," she said, pointing a shaking finger at John and me. "He says 'No,' and that woman just turns away."

I realized, suddenly, I was too exhausted to respond . . . even more, too tired to cry.

22

The Very Best Christmas Ever

Push it down.

That had been my refrain so many times when my father was ill. When things got overwhelming witnessing his cruel and progressive decline from Alzheimer's, I employed a desperate approach to cope. The mantra worked like this: I took my anguish and squashed it into a little imaginary box and then moved the box to a different place in my mind, to be opened only when I had more strength to bear it.

Now, two days after my mother's accident, I needed to do it again: get the box out and stuff all my feelings of despair into it, pushing them down, affixing a lid, and shoving it to the far reaches of my brain—letting it hover there, unopened, until things settled down and made more sense.

Because little made sense. We had lived through the TIA, prepared for my mother's homecoming, and let ourselves dream that perhaps we might have a "normal" Christmas after all, with a lot to celebrate. The girls had two weeks of winter vacation from school and the city was aglow with the little white lights strung on trees and buildings throughout the town. We needed to get a Christmas tree and a few presents (forget the Christmas cards) and relax after the crisis had passed. But now there was a new crisis. And nothing was normal.

The doctor said that my mother's fractured spine as well as her broken ribs made for a serious situation as she was not breathing deeply, which could lead to complications of pneumonia. Respiratory therapists worked to give her a "spirometer" to practice taking deep breaths and help expand her lungs, but my mother complained it hurt too much to inhale.

Suffering severe pain from her injury, she was drugged up with Vicodin. She knew who I was ... kind of ... but she also thought my father was still alive.

143

"Where's George? Why doesn't he ever come to see me?" she whimpered several times a day.

Worse, she needed twenty-four-hour surveillance to make sure she didn't try to get up and walk by herself. She couldn't ambulate more than a few shuffled steps, but in her addled mental state, she thought she could walk and attempted to get up to go to the bathroom several times a day, even to the point of sticking her legs through the hospital bed rails. Alonzo had caught her three times climbing out of bed just before she fell, and John had averted disaster twice. Even I had stopped her from falling once. All of us shuddered to think what would have happened if we had not been there.

"The situation with your mother is uncertain," said the neurologist, later in the week. "Will her pain reduce, her broken back heal? It should. It will just take time. Will she suffer a step down? Likely. Will she need a wheelchair to get around from here forward? Maybe. As I told you at the beginning, prepare yourself for the ride. It's a rodeo, and you're on a bronco."

Neurologists always seemed to talk in riddles, I thought.

After the doctor left, Alonzo arrived to stay the day. It was all I could do to create a schedule to have someone with my mom at all times. Inez stepped in to help too, along with Alonzo's niece, Mariana, who had moved to Portland from San Salvador in the past year. Mariana had met my mother on several occasions and, when she heard about the situation from Inez, generously offered to take some shifts to watch over my mother when we couldn't be there. Her kindness only reinforced the tremendous sense of gratitude I felt for the Mendez family.

"Momma mia," said Alonzo, staring at my mother, whose eyes were open but not comprehending. "She still doesn't know me."

"Nor me," I said, "most of the time."

"I'm so glad to find you both here," said Jan, the social worker, stepping brusquely into the room without knocking and taking us by surprise. "I'm here to let you know it's been all arranged."

"What's arranged?"

Jan's eyes would not meet ours. "It's difficult because of the holidays, you know. I have been on the phone for hours. Your mom was rejected at two places, but I finally got her into Soothing Breezes Nursing Home and Care Center. They're expecting her."

"Oh," I said, feeling virtually nothing. "When?"

"Today."

"Today? You've got to be kidding!" I cried.

"I'll be back shortly with her discharge papers for you to sign."

"Look at her! How can you move her, in this condition? Do the doctors know?"

Jan smiled a little condescendingly. "Yes, the doctors know. Everything has been approved. Your mother's insurance won't allow her to stay in the hospital any longer. Of course, she needs additional care. They'll do that at Soothing Breezes. Transport will be here at 2:15."

"That's only in a few hours!"

"That's how it works," said Jan, turning to leave.

Alonzo was shaking his head. "Momma mia! I don't like that woman!"

It was entirely too reminiscent of the rapid-fire hospital send-off my father was forced to comply with after his broken hip. "I'll make sure to take her drug list with me," I said, remembering the fiasco that nearly killed my father. I didn't know whether to be furious or terrified.

"She still can't breathe!" observed Alonzo. He had a way of stating the obvious that wasn't always helpful. "Doesn't Margaret have pneumonia? I don't like this."

"I'm not sure if it's pneumonia. The nurse said her lung sounds were a little rattly," I replied, not knowing exactly what that meant. Did a little rattly mean she had pneumonia? A little pneumonia? A lot? "She's on antibiotics," I added.

"No good. I don't like this," he grumbled again.

I picked up the phone to call John and tell him the turn of events when the kind physical therapist who had tended my mother through her TIA poked his head into the room. "May I?" he asked, wondering whether he could come in.

"I just heard," he said, with a pained expression. He walked over to my mother, who glanced at him like she had never seen him before.

"How can they push her out of here? Like this!" I queried, anxiously.

"There's not much they can do for a broken back," the therapist replied, but his voice was consoling. "Her kinds of fractures usually heal on their own . . . in time." He leaned down, closer to my mother. "Remember me? We were a good team! I came to wish you good luck!"

My mother stared into space. The therapist didn't appear to notice but only looked sad. His kindness was in such stark contrast to everything else this morning that I could feel tears forming in my eyes.

"Merry Christmas," he said, gently, with a slight squeeze to her hand, before turning to leave.

Pushing it down didn't work this time. I formed the box in my mind, but the lid didn't fit tightly enough. The feelings escaped, and so did the tears, and when Jan came back with the paperwork a few minutes later, they were coursing down my face.

Soothing Breezes was thirty minutes farther from our home than the hospital, which meant added time and inconvenience. Aside from the grave disappointment that my mother wouldn't be able to return home for Christmas, I also felt pulled in a thousand directions. Emily and Jennifer were home for the holidays, and I yearned to spend time with them—to try to pretend a sense of normalcy that wasn't there—but my mother was disoriented and needed someone with her for her own safety. Once again, we were in a time of crisis.

Mariana, thankfully, offered to stay the nights at Soothing Breezes. But each morning when I arrived, the heavy, dark bags under her brown eyes revealed that her stint was anything but "soothing." I wondered, in fact, whether she even slept.

"Your mother asked to go to the bathroom only eleven times last night," reported Mariana, evincing her gentle patience. "That's much better," she smiled weakly, "than the two nights before that, when she got up thirteen times."

This scenario could not go on much longer, or Mariana would be a new Soothing Breezes resident herself.

"Why do you think she does that?" I asked, "and can't she just go in her diaper?"

Mariana shook her head. "She doesn't like her diaper and wants it off at night. I want to honor her wishes."

Her words made me realize my own impatience, and I felt correspondingly guilty. I asked the nursing staff whether they had any ideas, and they said no. Mariana was obviously exhausted. I told her to go home; I would see her tonight at eleven and spend the entire day here. Alonzo, I knew, wouldn't be coming in to spell me today or for the next few days. He needed time with Inez and their family to get ready for Christmas—which was tomorrow.

Pulling out my journal, I settled down in the chair while my mother slept. But I couldn't write. Rather, I stared at the linoleum floor, feeling sorry for myself.

A nursing home is not a festive place to spend Christmas. A side of me wished it were already over. I had not had time to buy any presents. Our home was only minimally decorated. Everything this year was frazzled, last minute, and the closer Christmas got, the more inadequate I felt. I was also lonely—for John and the girls. But then I would remember that my mother was my family. And feel guilty all over again.

Before I left this morning, Jennifer told me I looked tired. She asked, would I *ever* be home?

Until my mother became more coherent, it didn't appear likely. There was too much risk. While her lung congestion was getting better, her orientation was not. Dr. Moore was growing concerned. Talking with him yesterday, he said he wondered whether the opiates she was on for pain were the culprits—augmenting a befuddled mental state.

Dr. Moore explained that some people, especially as they aged, displayed adverse reactions to narcotics and even to Vicodin. Sometimes painkillers could make rational older individuals appear as if they were suffering from dementia or even a stroke. To test his hunch, he immediately removed all opiates from my mother's copious drug list and prescribed only Tylenol for pain. He said it might take a day or two, but he hoped for some improvement.

All I could see so far today, though, was an increase in her discomfort and back pain. All she wanted to do was lie in bed, feeling too uncomfortable to leave her room and too tired from being up all night with her stream of trips to the bathroom.

That was okay with me; I didn't wish to leave the room anyway. I found Soothing Breezes overwhelmingly depressing. The food was yucky; the nurses on a mission to get things done; there was no place to go to escape. I especially wished to avoid the dining area. Once more, I felt transported back to the Land of the Pink Bibs. They were everywhere. The little neck aprons were obviously the uniform of choice for all nursing home residents anywhere in the world. And it was beginning to frighten me that every pink-bibbed patient I had come across at Montavilla and now at Soothing Breezes seemed to have a startling resemblance to one another—the way their heads were canted or how they drooped in their wheelchairs.

The fact that it was Christmas only made everything worse. As the hours dragged on and my mood deteriorated, I found myself wondering, did grinches steal Christmas or did grinches hate Christmas? I knew, with only a little bit more prodding, I could very easily become one. What's more, I could write the operating manual for grinches.

If I were a grinch and wanted to make Christmas truly miserable for everyone, the easiest thing would be to put people in a nursing home, in a hospital bed, in a brown room with one overhead fluorescent light that made your skin turn green, and with no decorations whatsoever. Then, take away anything that could let your thoughts take flight, like TV, music, or books. (There was no TV here.) Add some people moaning next door to you, and sprinkle the room with fear and urine smells.

To embezzle Christmas, a grinch's dream was Soothing Breezes.

"May I come in for a minute?"

It was the nurse's aide, Lily, who had been tending to my mother for the past two days. Small boned and petite, with shiny, dark hair and pale skin, she seemed too small to be able to manage some of the heftier patients. Her voice was distinctive—kind, with a hint of a lilt. Her name seemed to fit her, for she reminded me of a wildflower.

"Oh, hi. Sure."

"How is your mother this afternoon?"

"Sleeping mostly. She was up eleven times last night."

"I know. I came in a few times to help out your caregiver." Lily walked over to stand by my mother, who fluttered her eyes open. "My shift is over now, Margaret, and I'm going home," she said, smiling. Then, she turned toward me.

"I've noticed you and your family have been here a lot; it's obvious you really care about your mother."

I tried veiling the grinch expression on my face.

"I know you can't leave her alone," she continued.

"I need to go to the bathroom," my mother suddenly groaned, grabbing at the bed rail.

"Let me," jumped in Lily, who immediately proved her strength. She knew precisely where all the bed rail buttons were, whereas I still had problems locating the right ones, often moving my mother's head when I meant to move her feet. Lily had the bars down in a flash. She aided my mother to a sitting position, placed the walker next to the bed, and helped her stand and grip the handles. Placing her arm round my mother's waist, they both shuffled like a pair of turtles toward the bathroom.

Once back and safely in bed, Lily repositioned my mother's bed rails, locking them in place. "I wonder if you'd let me do something for you?" she asked, while tucking my mother in the sheets.

"Um, what?"

Lily turned her brown eyes on me. "I would like to sit with your mother tomorrow morning, on Christmas Day, so you can have that time with your family."

I was unable to speak for a moment.

She went right on. "I celebrate Christmas on Christmas Eve with my family. I don't work tomorrow; I have it off. There is nothing I would like more than to be with your mother Christmas morning so that you can be home with your husband and girls."

Lily didn't wait for a reply, but I couldn't have given her one anyway. The lump was too great in the back of my throat. "Good; I'll be here at eight o'clock then," she said with a happy smile. "Enjoy your beautiful family."

The aide had flitted out the door before I could pull my wits together. What had just happened? I thought, stunned. An almost total stranger had just given me the most gracious Christmas gift I'd ever received in my life. I jumped up to thank her, but Lily had already disappeared by the time I reached the hallway.

"I like that girl," said my mother, looking at the door.

"Yes," I replied. One simple gesture had just transformed Christmas. "I do too."

But soon something else was about to turn Soothing Breezes on its head.

Not long after Lily had left, a commotion started brewing down the corridor. At first, it didn't register. It was the sound of laughter—something not often heard in nursing homes. Pausing to listen, I recognized those voices...

"Happy Early Christmas, Nana!" shouted Emily and Jennifer, bursting into the room. Between them, they carried a four-foot-high artificial tree. They also lugged brown paper bags overflowing with wrapped presents, red decorating balls, strings of little white lights, and an extension cord. Behind them, John was trying to maneuver a small TV from Nana's house.

"Why, what's this?" my mother said, reaching out to hug and kiss them all. "Emily, Jennifer, what have you done?" Her cognizance startled me nearly as much as the holiday parade.

Emily spoke first. "Well, Dad, Jennifer, and I were talking at breakfast that we thought Mom looked tired and so did you, and no one seemed much in the Christmas spirit. We decided we needed to do something about it. If you can't be home for Christmas, we thought we would bring it here—to you!"

"You bought a tree?" I asked John.

"Well, there has to be a tree, even if it is artificial!" offered Jennifer. "It just wouldn't be Christmas without one. We also brought Papa's boom box and some Christmas CDs."

"That's lovely," said my mother, really smiling for the first time since her fall. It was like she suddenly woke up.

"It'll be a party, like we used to do for Papa," said Emily.

"We're going to really rock and roll and shake up this place," said John.

I knew, of course, he didn't really mean it, but before long, the sad little nursing home room was transfigured to resemble a storefront window. The girls tacked the white lights around. John set up the tree and plugged in the small lights to illuminate it. Emily and Jennifer trimmed the green, bushy branches with bright red balls. Soon the CD player hummed with the caroling of Nat King Cole. Before long, nurses, aides, and even other patients stopped by to see what the merriment was about and to admire the decorations.

"Merry Christmas," my mother said at least a dozen times, for the cheer was contagious.

"Wait 'til tomorrow, Nana," said Emily, sitting on my mother's bed. "We're going to bring Christmas dinner here and take over a meeting room. Dad already asked, and they said it's okay because no one will be there tomorrow. It will be the best Christmas ever!"

"Ooh, that sounds fun," chirped Nana, squeezing her hand and then reaching out to squeeze Jennifer's and mine.

John was busy pouring eggnog in plastic cups and passing it around. The door opened, and a night nurse poked her head in. He offered her a glass. She refused.

Taking in the room full of lights, the twinkling tree, the TV, and the CD player sending out Christmas music, she frowned.

"You've got a heck o' a lot of stuff goin' on in here," she said, shaking her head. "I just hope you don't blow the fuse."

23

Three Things

*W*hen my mother continued becoming weaker physically while at the same time improving mentally, I began growing suspicious. Two trajectories appeared to be going on at once: one, increasing lucidity, which was cause to rejoice, but two, declining mobility. Her physical strength seemed so diminished I wondered whether she would ever walk on her own, without the aid of a wheelchair, again.

Soothing Breezes vociferously proclaimed that my mother was receiving the best physical therapy available with at least one session with a licensed therapist daily. Alonzo, who was back after Christmas and sat with my mother during the day, claimed he never saw it happen. It was possible that it occurred at exactly the time that Alonzo would take his fifteen-minute breaks, but my mother, too, said she couldn't remember having therapy, although her memory was a bit more unreliable. Yet I began doubting that she was actually receiving it and asked personnel.

"See, it's checked off on the door," said the staff worker. "When they come by, they mark it off on this paper."

Alonzo was shaking his head. "I was here then. No one came by the room."

"Well, it's checked off," she replied, coolly.

"*Who* checked it off?" continued Alonzo.

"The therapist. At two o'clock. It says right there."

"No therapist was here at two o'clock today. I know that."

The woman shrugged. "All I can say is that it has been checked off. Maybe you were sleeping or weren't here."

Alonzo was on the verge of losing his temper. He took great pride in his veracity and attention to his duties. "Well, I could check things off, too, see!"

he exclaimed, after the staff person had left. He pretended to take a pencil and check-check-check the sheet that hung on the inside of my mother's door. "No one has showed up to do therapy, except for one time."

Alonzo went back to his chair and sat down in a huff. I felt more resigned. Insurance was running out for my mother's nursing home stay, but everyone was anxious to get her home anyway. The trouble was, there was no more insurance for physical therapy once she got home. According to Medicare regulations, she had had as much therapy as appropriate for her level of disability. In other words, she had progressed as far as she could go in terms of rehab. Yet it seemed so shortsighted. She came into the hospital walking; she left the hospital needing a wheelchair.

My mother felt dizzy when she rose up in bed. After three weeks, we had all learned how to transfer her to the wheelchair, but she hated it.

"I'll never be able to walk out and see those little lambs in the barn again," she said, sounding depressed. But it was more than just walking through the field. Her sorrow derived from fear. Her legs felt too weak to hold her, she confided, and she was frightened she would fall again. "The only good thing is that I won't have to exercise anymore," she said, finding something positive in her darkening world.

The social worker at Soothing Breezes was pragmatic when we discussed my mother's home situation. "How is she going to navigate the stairs in her house?" she asked. "She may remain in her wheelchair for the rest of her life."

"Can't she improve if she works at it?"

"In our experience, considering her age and lack of mobility, by only a fraction. Perhaps it's time you thought about moving your mom to an assisted living situation, where there are no stairs to contend with. Soothing Breezes has a lovely new building that has three levels of care, depending on personal need. Would you like us to arrange a tour for you and your mother?"

My mother, when I brought up the subject, was adamant. "I want to go home."

My sisters, who lived out of town, were not so sure. They wondered how long she could manage living in her large home, with only Alonzo and Inez and sometimes Mariana. They were pessimistic. A teenage niece was even more frank.

"She should move. She *is* old."

Emily and Jennifer disagreed. "Nana loves her home. I think she can get better."

So did Inez and Alonzo.

"Your momma has a big fighting spirit," said Alonzo. "I don't think we should give up on her. Don't you know anybody else who could help?"

Dr. Moore didn't have any ideas. He said he already had had several run-ins with my mother's insurance. He speculated that physical therapy might still be appropriate, but even he could get nowhere with Medicare. She was caught in an unfortunate window: not bad enough from suffering a severe stroke, which would allow her to qualify for more therapy, but not good enough to recover on her own without it.

This time, no one was talking about celebrations getting my mother home. Realistically, we all knew it was going to be a trial in itself. School had started up again for the girls, John was busy at work, the holidays were over, my writing career was going badly, and Soothing Breezes was not encouraging about my mother's prognosis. She still was not sleeping well—waking up often in the night, asking to go to the bathroom. A recipe for falling.

Pairing getting used to a wheelchair existence with poor sleeping habits, as well as worsening vision, my mother's spirits, too, seemed to be on the decline.

"It's quite normal for older people to be depressed and not sleep well," said the social worker. "It's the norm."

"What can we do about it?" I asked.

"Not much," was her realistic but unhelpful reply.

The wheelchair was an armload getting up and down the outside steps, and I began worrying that Alonzo would be the next one to have an accident. My mother, with help, could still navigate getting up and down, but with her weakening quadriceps, I wondered how much longer that would be possible.

"You're a happy bunch," said John, coming home from work one evening and finding Emily, Jennifer, and me discussing the situation. Both the girls were admonishing me for giving up; and it was true, to a point. When John stepped in, my head was cradled in my arms on the table.

"I think it really may be time to move Mom from the house," I admitted, knowing I was at last defeated.

"What does *she* want?" asked John.

"You know. She wants to stay in her own home. But that's getting really hard."

"What about calling Sarah?" he said, handing me a glass of wine.

The thought had not crossed my mind before. Sarah Harris was a friend who was also a physical therapist. She had worked as the lead physical therapist at a large hospital in Portland for nearly twenty years. She was an expert in pain management, but I didn't know much more about what she did.

"You might ask her her thoughts about your mom," said John, "before you throw out the baby with the bathwater."

I highly doubted that Sarah would be able to say much that was different from everyone else, but it was worth a try. If she were also discouraging, then I would take steps to look at other living arrangements.

Surprisingly, what she advised was the exact opposite of all the other advice I'd received. Sarah said new advances in physical therapy were showing highly positive results when it came to neurological disorders. Some newer treatments, such as Feldenkrais, in which Sarah was also certified, were very helpful when teamed with traditional therapies. She said she had a friend and professional colleague, Elizabeth Ross, who was a licensed therapist, also certified in Feldenkrais, who might be able to come to my mother's home on a private basis a few times a week.

"Think of it like paying for your mom to have a personal trainer, for a while. I wouldn't give up on her."

Initially, my mother was reluctant. She was beginning to feel safe in the wheelchair and rapidly losing not only all the strength in her quads, but what remained of her confidence in walking. But after the first visit with Elizabeth, all that changed. As we observed when she walked in the door for the first time, Elizabeth was a gentle soul and a beautiful human being. Before the first session was over, my mother was captivated. And the feeling, for Elizabeth, was mutual. The bond that developed between them was to last throughout the rest of their lives.

Gently, with baby steps, Elizabeth taught my mother a few simple exercises to begin with to try to build up some muscles in her legs. Next she started work on balance. She carefully explained how my mother could safely transfer herself from a bed to a chair or from a chair to standing up. When my mother complained of dizziness, Elizabeth had an answer.

"It's perfectly normal to feel dizzy after you've been lying down and then attempt to sit up. Remember to always sit on the side of the bed for a while before you stand up. I'll say it again: *always sit for a while on the side of the bed to get your bearings before you try to stand up.* You may want to pop right up (my mother laughed; she never popped up) but don't, Margaret. Get some nice oxygen to your brain first. Then stand up."

"But I can't stand up by myself," my mother proclaimed. "Someone needs to lift me up."

"You will," said Elizabeth.

The therapist came two times a week at first and instructed Alonzo and me about her exercise regime. Leg lifts. Quadriceps training. Bicep curls. Tai chi stuff. And more.

My mother never relished it but didn't want to disappoint Elizabeth.

"You may never walk again without a walker, Margaret," said Elizabeth after a couple of weeks, "but you *will* walk. I believe you will be able to put that wheelchair back in the closet or send it back wherever you rented it."

Four months later, when the grip of rain was letting up and cherry trees were beginning to blossom along the city streets, my mother had a follow-up visit with her internist, Dr. Moore. Time had been healing; her back had repaired, and so had her ribs. There had been no repeat of TIA episodes. The physician admitted being amazed at her progress.

My mother was noticeably pleased by his words, especially when he called her "frisky." But it was apparent that something was still troubling her. With a little prodding, she finally admitted it to her doctor.

"I am kind of worried, well, very worried actually, about a small leg tremor I have on occasion."

"You're concerned it may be Parkinson's?" asked Dr. Moore, astutely.

"Yes." Her voice got more quiet. "And I'm also worried that I might get . . . Alzheimer's."

Dr. Moore's expression was not condescending but serious. He came closer to her and looked her squarely in the face.

"I think every older person has those same anxieties," he acknowledged. Then he said something that my mother kept close to her all her life. I never knew whether it was actually true or not, but it didn't really matter. It was a fact that gave her hope, and she never let it go.

"I don't mean to offend you, Margaret, but you are too old to get Parkinson's or Alzheimer's disease. You'd either have them by now or not. The tremor is most likely caused by the recent urinary tract infection you just had. It should go away in time."

After his words, some of the depression my mother evinced ever since her first TIA, six months before, began to recede. I realized I had never been cognizant of how much fear of developing Alzheimer's had been dragging down her psyche. Yet the change in her outlook was palpable. Coming to our house for dinner later that week, she seemed positively gay. She chatted with Emily about her summer job plans and talked enthusiastically about Jennifer's upcoming eighth-grade graduation, which she planned to attend—with no need of a wheelchair.

"Dr. Moore was right," my mother announced between bites of salmon. "There *are* some good things about getting as old as I am. He said there were two. But actually, there are three."

"What are they, Nana?" asked Emily.

"Well, I can't get Parkinson's and I can't get Alzheimer's."

"That's good," agreed Jennifer. "But what's the third?"

My mother smiled.

"I can't get pregnant."

What I Wish I'd Known

The Art to Aging Healthfully for Your Body and Your Mind

Elizabeth Eckstrom, MD, MPH, MACP

*M*argaret mentioned that there were three good things about getting old. In reality, there are lots more than three, but much depends upon a person having the knowledge of the "dos and don'ts" of aging well. This chapter reveals the latest research on several key factors to successful aging:

1. How to promote longevity
2. How to achieve quality of life
3. How to maintain good brain function
4. The importance of continuing community involvement
5. Why creativity regenerates the mind and body

Each of these categories is essential to aging healthfully. And each requires some personal effort and commitment. But by taking control of your aging—armed with the understanding of ways to achieve better outcomes—you have the opportunity to make a real difference in how you age. Instead of greeting age with fear, you can meet it like a friend—with active engagement and a determination to make it positive—and, yes, even find joy and inspiration in the process.

So what are scientists discovering about healthy aging? And what do *you* need to know to successfully chart your own course? Let's look specifically at five important questions researchers are investigating and the fascinating answers that are arising.

WHAT IS LONGEVITY AND
WHAT CAN I DO TO PROMOTE IT?

Longevity is how long we live. Most of us want to live as long as we can, but with a caveat: we don't want to be disabled. Is there anything we can do to help us live longer and maintain our health?

Yes, and it boils down to a simple mantra: *Practice a healthy lifestyle!* Several points are key in carrying this out:

- Engaging in regular exercise
- Eating a healthy Mediterranean diet, full of fruits and vegetables
- Avoiding smoking
- Drinking no more than one alcoholc drink per day if over sixty-five
- Wearing your seatbelt—always—when in the car
- Maintaining an ideal body weight

Research shows that longevity and healthy living are inextricably linked. In a landmark study by Yates and colleagues, it was documented that men adhering to a healthy lifestyle at age seventy had a significantly better chance of reaching ninety than those following a less healthy life-style. Believe it or not, 54 percent of the seventy-year-olds who regularly exercised, didn't smoke, and didn't have obesity, diabetes, or high blood pressure, lived to ninety years old—and that was men! However, for those men who practiced fewer of the essential elements, the chances of achieving older age dropped considerably. Yates's study showed that when seventy-year-old men participated in only two healthful habits, just 30 percent of them made it to ninety. Even more noteworthy, for those men who practiced none of the healthy behaviors, a mere *4 percent lived to be ninety years old.*

In another study, Khaw and colleagues documented that exercise, moderate alcohol intake, eating enough fruits and vegetables, and not smoking were critical elements to achieving longevity. Their research demonstrated that people who practiced all four healthful behaviors, as compared to those who did none, lived fourteen years longer! Further, the impact of healthy choices on mortality was greater for those over sixty-five years than those under sixty-five.

So if you want to live longer, be sure you are practicing an all-around healthy lifestyle!

HOW DO I ACHIEVE A GOOD QUALITY OF LIFE AS I AGE?

Most of us want to live a long time, but we don't want that time to be spent in a wheelchair, or in a nursing home, or suffering from end-stage dementia. Our preference would be to live a healthy life for as long as we can and then die quickly. Who wouldn't wish to be perfectly healthy until reaching one hundred and then die peacefully in their sleep? Well, Dr. James Fries at Stanford University has researched and written extensively on the notion of "compression of morbidity"—or, in simpler terms, the concept of living longer and well and *compressing* any disabled time (*morbidity*) into the smallest possible time before death.

Fries's research joins other studies documenting that there is *one* best way to achieve this goal. And while many of you, like Margaret, may be getting sick of hearing it, it is the most valuable tool in maintaining a quality of life and a compression of disability.

Daily exercise.

Like Fries, numerous scientists are discovering that exercise plays a pivotal role in how well you age. By following the exercise recommendations I have outlined throughout this book, you *can* make a real difference in the quality of your life and, as you age, greatly reduce the amount of time spent not being able to care for yourself.

WHAT CAN I DO TO MAINTAIN (OR EVEN IMPROVE) GOOD BRAIN FUNCTION AS I GET OLDER?

In previous chapters, I have talked a lot about dementia and what it means to have cognitive decline. I have not yet discussed ways to *prevent it*. Yet people who do not have cognitive impairment are far more likely to succeed at healthy aging. Therefore, protecting your brain is one of the most important things you can do to age well! That being said, how do you do it?

Neuroscientists are finding that you can do some important things to help shield your brain from aging's deleterious effects and to aid in its healthy functioning. Among these, three are the chart toppers:

1. *Exercise for at least thirty minutes daily.*

(Here we go again! Refer to the chapters on exercise for recommendations.)

2. *Follow a Mediterranean diet.*

Studies are documenting that people who adhere to the Mediterranean diet have a marked decrease in heart problems, dementia, and many other medical tribulations as they age. It is a diet that you can follow for the rest of your life, because when you learn how to do it, it doesn't feel like dieting. It feels good!

- Your diet should hinge on fresh fruits and vegetables. *Get five colors every day*! For example, spinach, tomatoes, peaches, blueberries, oranges or squash. Focus on the "low glycemic load" fruits and vegetables; these are the ones with less sugar in them. All of the ones listed above are low glycemic load, as are all other berries, apricots, cantaloupe, green beans, kale, yams, peppers, onions, broccoli, cauliflower, and brussels sprouts. But remember, hold off on the ranch dressing. Rather, try roasting vegetables in the oven in a little olive oil and fennel seed.
- Try to avoid high-sugar fruits and vegetables. These include corn, peas, watermelon, cherries, pineapple, grapes, and potatoes. Eat these in much smaller quantities.
- Eat lots of whole grains and legumes, lentils, beans, whole-grain bread, and other whole-grain items. For a treat, try a piece of toasted Dave's Killer Bread (developed in the Northwest—or look around for a similar healthy bread in your area) with almond butter on it for breakfast.
- Eat healthy oils such as olive and canola oil. Healthy fats include almonds, walnuts, and avocados—all especially good for you.
- Your protein, other than beans, should be derived mostly from fish and chicken breast. Cook it on the grill or under the broiler. (No frying in hot oil!) You may eat nonfat cottage cheese and yogurt, as both are healthy and delicious when paired with berries. Also, you can add some tuna fish and tomatoes to the cottage cheese for a super healthy lunch.
- Do not eat red meat more than twice a month. If you eat red meat, it should be low-fat varieties and in small-sized portions.
- Do not eat butter, ice cream, cheese, or sweets. You may drink coffee without sugar or cream (but it is okay to add nonfat milk).
- You may have one to two ounces of dark chocolate daily. This is your treat. But don't eat it right before bed as it has some caffeine.

3. *Learn new things!*

Exciting new research is showing that challenging your brain to *become skilled at something new* is one of the best ways to maintain its function. Learn a new language or take up playing a new musical instrument. These techniques can help expand your social horizons. Even more, groundbreaking research is revealing that both of these skills can *help your brain cells regenerate*—or grow and repair damage incurred from getting older.

Even better: you don't have to become the next Emanuel Ax or André Watts to revitalize your brain. If learning music or trying out a different instrument is new for you, even learning simple tunes like "Twinkle, Twinkle, Little Star" can help jump-start your brain to repair and make new cells.

HOW DO I STAY ACTIVELY ENGAGED IN MY COMMUNITY AS I GET OLDER, AND IS IT IMPORTANT?

Yes, it is important. Staying involved in cultural, educational, and civic activities is a critical aspect of healthy aging. It provides for better physical, mental, and cognitive health as well as beneficial social integration. Moreover, it is an economic asset rather than a drain on the system. However, it is not always easy for people to continue to stay engaged in their community as they age. This is highly unfortunate.

Think about it: Older adults have a wealth of wisdom and practical knowledge to share with the younger people in our communities. Also, as we age, our perspective broadens, allowing us to see life from differing points of view. These attributes of older adults make them an amazing resource to our communities—if only we could readily tap into it.

Here lies the rub: often, younger people do not recognize the value of spending time with older people, and those older folks have difficulty getting out. What happens? They end up becoming stuck at home. This can lead to a downhill spiral—feelings of loneliness, isolation, and lack of self-worth. These are not only negatives for them . . . but for society at large as well.

Marcy's parents were very active and connected with family, friends, and work for many years. When they were less able to get out they were lucky to have Emily and Jennifer (plus all of Inez's and Alonzo's family for many years) and lunches with Marcy to keep them engaged in life. This sense of being a valued and contributing member is essential to maintaining cognition and preventing depression and functional dependence.

WHAT ARE WE LEARNING ABOUT THE VALUE OF BEING CREATIVE AS WE AGE?

Attempting creative pursuits is shown to be strongly correlated with positive and healthy outcomes as we age. Building new skills, partaking in hobbies, and engaging in creative activities all require the brain to remodel itself. This function jump-starts growth of new brain cells acting to replace those that are growing older or have become damaged.

Recent studies have shown that older individuals who have been involved in weekly participatory art programs have demonstrated over a two-year interval:

- Better health, fewer doctor visits, and less medication usage
- More positive responses on mental health measures
- More involvement in overall activities

Interestingly, even people with a beginning dementia are able to create with the support of the group. In one study, when residents of a dementia care facility were encouraged to participate in storytelling, this led to more smiling and greeting of others, engaging in conversations, and humming. Patients fell asleep more easily, had less agitated behaviors such as wandering and repetitive shouting, and required less assistance with things like going to the bathroom.

Now you can see why arts activities and *The Airplane Diaries* were so important to Dr. Cottrell.

In essence, there are many things we can all do to promote healthy aging—for our loved ones and for ourselves. It is never too early—or too late—to begin. And you don't have to be completely disease-free to "qualify" for good aging; people who suffer from illnesses such as cancer, diabetes, heart problems, or numerous other ailments can still age successfully—physically, mentally, and emotionally—by making the best of their situation and following the guidelines above.

It boils down to a fork in the road and the path you choose. There are two before you. You can decide to let *age* take the lead and run its own decelerating course in its own fashion. Or you can choose to sign up, pin on the running bib, and actively engage in the race. Aging is a marathon of sorts. But plenty of eighty- and ninety-year-olds today can be found running marathons.

So I encourage you to take that other path. Run the race! Play the piano! Take a painting class! Volunteer at the library!

And the result? *Thrive.*

24

I See Little Green Men

"*Getting* old is not for sissies," said my mother when I picked her up to take her to an appointment with the eye doctor.

It was true. Last week she'd been to the audiologist to check her hearing aids. The week before it was to her dentist because of an aching tooth that, most likely, would have to be pulled. Then there were the visits to the cardiologist to monitor her atrial fibrillation and mild congestive heart failure; to the urologist to keep up with bladder problems that she'd developed since her TIA; to the internist to prescribe medicine for nausea, dizziness, sleeping, and an underactive thyroid; and now to the ophthalmologist. The result was a medication list that continued expanding longer and longer, like an ever-lengthening paper chain.

Each doctor was treating a part of my mother, but I never felt certain who was looking after the whole person. It almost seemed medical care for an old person was akin to patching up Humpty Dumpty—all the king's horses and all the king's men were trying to put the pieces of my mother together again. Often I found myself wishing I could assemble the different specialists on a panel where I could ask questions of them. Together they could also discuss among themselves the composite parts and build an entire portrait of my mother that we could all understand.

But that was unlikely. The real truth was that there was never enough time during the visits to ask a lot of questions. I didn't blame the physicians; I respected most of them and knew, in today's healthcare world, they were under the gun to see lots of patients. That meant *I* had to be the one to try to pull the disparate picture together, which meant asking questions.

Some doctors were more welcoming of queries than others. Some, like the ophthalmologist we were seeing today—a physician distinguished for his work with macular degeneration—were not. With countless research and clinical demands on his time, he had little patience for inconsequential chit-chat. He had made that clear on previous visits when I hoped to discuss some things I'd researched on the Internet. When I posed questions, he came back with his own for me:

"Where did you hear *that*?"

"Where did you get *that* figure?"

"Just what *are* you trying to say?"

"So what is your *question*?"

After that, I was usually too intimidated to continue.

Today, though, was different. Today I had a firm list of questions I really wanted answers to. I could tell my mother's vision was worse, even with some newer treatments. Not being able to read was making her miserable. And I knew she wasn't alone.

Macular degeneration is relatively common in old people. It is the leading cause of blindness in older adults. A friend, who was a physician, told me that when people receive the diagnosis of macular degeneration, it could be as devastating as being told they have cancer. Like the loss of other important senses, the threat of blindness looming was terrifying. Losing the ability to see or hear effectively shrank their world, leaving them with feelings of isolation, vulnerability, and being cut off from life.

As I feared, the doctor gave my mother the news that the visudyne treatments she'd been getting to curtail the progression of macular degeneration were not succeeding. He was willing to try them a few more times, but the prognosis wasn't good. All he could recommend was low-vision aids.

Her face fell. I knew she was too disappointed to speak, so I asked the questions for her. I had them jotted down in my notebook so as not to forget the important ones.

"Are there any other treatments that we might try? What were the results of the florescene angiogram? Are the blood vessels behind her eyes still leaking? Does she have wet or dry macular degeneration? Is there a difference between the two? Does it usually happen to both eyes at once, like Mom's? Should she continue with the eye drops? What can she do now?"

The doctor, who already had one foot out the door, for he had many more patients to see and was already far behind, was terse in his responses. I wrote them next to my questions. "Not really. Leakage. Yes. Wet. No. Sometimes. Yes. Not much."

There wasn't much left to make the answers worse, so I blurted out the one question that my mother had confided to me, knowing she was going to kill me.

"Why is my mother seeing little green men?"

As soon as the words were out of my mouth I regretted it. Now the doctor would think not only was my mother a psychiatric patient, but I was, too.

"You're seeing little green men?" he asked, taking his foot from the doorjamb and stepping back inside the room.

My mother looked stricken. "I didn't want her to bring that up."

"When do you see these little green men, Margaret?"

"Only occasionally. *Rarely.*"

"Are these little green men real to you?"

"Real? Oh, no; they're not real. But I can see them just the same."

"Do you see other things? Maybe like policemen, or dwarves?"

Now my mother stared at him like he was losing his mind. "No, not policemen or dwarves."

"Anything else?" said the doctor. "Do you see anything else?"

"Flowers, sometimes," she said, sounding guilty.

"Are the flowers real?"

"No. They are pretty though. But I know they're not real."

"How long have you been seeing these little green men?"

My mother took a breath. "For about a year now."

"A year? Why haven't you told me?" I interrupted.

"I didn't want to upset you. And . . . I thought it was better not to talk about it."

"Because, Margaret, you are afraid of being considered insane," the doctor said.

Her ashamed expression revealed that was exactly what she thought—that she was going crazy.

"You are not losing your mind. You have classic Charles Bonnet syndrome."

"What kind of syndrome?" I asked.

"Is that . . . a disease?" said my mother.

The renowned and hurried doctor suddenly seemed remarkably patient.

"Charles Bonnet syndrome is not a disease. It's a condition that is very common in older patients who have severe macular degeneration. It's a trick of memory, somewhat reminiscent of the 'phantom arm syndrome.' When a person loses a limb, there are times when the mind still can 'feel' that limb, even though it isn't there. It's the same thing with Charles Bonnet. The brain creates hallucinogenic images—sometimes benign, sometimes quite peculiar, like little green men. The important thing is: You know they're not really there, even if you 'see' them."

The relief on my mother's face was profound. "I have been so worried! I thought I was losing my mind."

"How many people have this Charles Bonnet?" I asked.

"Studies show at least 15 percent. But in my practice, I'd say it's upward to 50 percent."

"Then why have we not heard about it before?"

"Because they don't teach doctors about it in medical school," said the doctor. "Most medical professionals, outside of eye specialists, have never heard of it, which is unfortunate. They leave their patients thinking the worst. If someone has the courage to bring it up to their general practitioner, their doctor will most likely diagnose it as a psychiatric problem or mental disease."

It struck me how much suffering must go on in old people who had Charles Bonnet syndrome. Along with losing their eyesight with macular degeneration, they thought, incorrectly, that they were losing their mind, too. Especially after having experienced a TIA, any kind of hallucination must be terrifying. It was probably the best news that this doctor had ever given my mother.

He patted her on her shoulder. He was going to give the visudyne therapy a few more tries. He told me he could give me some literature on Charles Bonnet if I wanted.

The poor doctor—he did something he had no intention of doing. He made me only want to ask more questions.

What I Wish I'd Known

Come to Your Senses! The Value of Aids

Elizabeth Eckstrom, MD, MPH, MACP

*H*ow many times have you seen a frail older woman walking down the sidewalk, gingerly placing her walker in front of her with each step? Though we can appreciate her tenacity, secretly we say to ourselves, "I will never let that happen to me! I would be too embarrassed to use a walker in public."

Well, one of the best pieces of advice I can possibly give you is this: *embrace aids as they help maintain independence.*

That doesn't mean that you should use a walker if you don't need one, but if your gait has declined from severe arthritis, a stroke, lowered vision, or loss of sensation in your feet from diabetes, a walker could mean all the difference between taking enjoyable outings or being stuck in your home all day.

If you find yourself reluctant to use aids, it's time to change your perspective. This chapter will explain some of the reasons they are so important and hopefully help ensure that you or your loved one has the right ones when you need them.

VISION AIDS

For whatever reason, glasses do not invoke the same negative stigma as many other types of aids—probably because so many young people need them. Corrective lenses are an incredibly valuable tool as we get older, and it is important to see your eye doctor at least yearly. But if there is one tip I can give about glasses, it is this: keep it simple.

Too often, many persons switch to bifocals or trifocals when they get older, considering them efficient. However, this can result in real problems. As we age, our eyes become less proficient at adjusting to multiple lenses, especially when we change the direction of our gaze quickly. When we step off a curb or walk down the stairs, it is easy for our eyes to accidentally look through the lower reading lenses, miss the step or crosswalk edge, and fall.

Studies have shown that you can prevent at least *one fall over the next year* if you conscientiously remove your bifocal lenses and put on your single-focal lenses when you move about. Better yet, steer completely clear of bifocals and trifocals when you are a little older. Rather, keep one pair of glasses for reading and the other for everything else.

Other problems can develop with vision over time. Marcy's mother had macular degeneration, which is one of the worst eye problems older people can get. Multivitamins can help slow vision decline, but nothing cures macular degeneration. For macular degeneration and other diseases that cause low vision, it is essential not just to make sure you have the right glasses, but to visit a low-vision clinic. Trained eye specialists can help you find aids—including magnifiers, telescopes, and video and computer devices—to give you back the best possible vision.

HEARING AIDS

I can't tell you how many times someone who had struggled to hear for years finally agreed to get hearing aids and spent a lot of money on them only to be thoroughly disappointed. They assumed the aids would help them hear better but discovered instead that the devices only seemed to amplify all noises without making them any clearer. Hearing aids are great at magnifying sound, but the problem is, they have little ability to pick out just the sounds you *want to hear*. So in a quiet room with just one person talking, hearing aids can be very useful, but in a noisy restaurant, you will hear all the background noises just as loudly as you hear the person speaking next to you, resulting in a frustrating experience.

Audiologists and ear, nose, and throat doctors ("ENTs") can help in these cases. Working with you, they can assist in making the aids function better for you, but it is tricky business and requires a lot of patience and frequent appointments to get things adjusted just right.

This being true, and understanding all the challenges associated with hearing aids, I cannot overemphasize the importance of good hearing to health. Studies have proved that decreased hearing is associated with an increased risk of mortality. Additionally, poorer hearing ability is also associated with an increased risk of memory decline. Therefore, investing in hearing aids and *making the effort to get the right ones adjusted for you* is very much worth it.

For those who can't afford hearing aids or who might have memory troubles that make hearing aids impossible to use, I recommend a handy device called a pocket amplifier. The simplest varieties of these have a small box with a microphone that one person speaks into, and the hearing-impaired person has headphones or an earbud that is attached to the same box and that allows the person to clearly hear the spoken words. Fancier versions have a microphone that one person wears around the neck and a *wireless* sound system—so that the hearing-impaired person wears only a small earbud. Naturally, these only work for two people, but they are great for using around the house rather than having to yell, and if the two of you go out to a noisy restaurant, they allow you to speak to each other without amplification of the background noise. Pocket amplifiers also work very well at doctor's appointments for those who are hard of hearing. I encourage all doctors' offices to have one available for their patients who have hearing difficulties.

GAIT AIDS

Repeatedly, we have shared in this book the most critical practice to aging well: regular exercise. Reduced mobility is one of the biggest threats to staying healthy; it is something to be avoided at all costs. But what do you do if walking is difficult, like it was for Marcy's mom? What if your loved one is unsteady, or falling occasionally, or feeling too tired to walk more than a few blocks?

Now is the time to get a gait aid.

Before beginning to use any type of gait aid, however, it is important to ask your doctor for a referral to a physical therapist for a gait and balance evaluation. A therapist can teach you exercises to improve your gait and muscle strength and also show you how to use the gait aid correctly.

Walking sticks are the simplest and least intrusive of the gait aids. They can help people remain independent for a very long time, particularly if they use them in both hands. I recommend getting good sturdy hiking sticks—also known as trekking poles—at a sporting goods store and using them for all walking.

A far more obvious gait aid is a walker. While admittedly more conspicuous than trekking poles, they also provide a lot more support. And today, walkers are much sleeker, more colorful, and more useful than they used to be. The best ones have wheels (good for anyone who doesn't have a movement disorder like Parkinson's disease), brakes, a seat (so that you can walk as far as you can, sit down and rest, and then walk some more), and a basket to carry items. Rather than a device that characterizes infirmity, think of it as a tool to uphold your independence.

HOME AIDS

Numerous aids are available that allow older people to function more independently and that help prevent accidents. In my opinion, a few rise to the top in usefulness. A device called a "reacher" can assist you in retrieving items from shelves or that drop on the floor. Stools specifically designed to sit in the shower or tub can reduce the threat of falls when bathing. Telephone amplifiers are great for those hard of hearing. Safety aids such as grab bars next to the toilet and raised toilet seats are practical and easy to install. Levered handles on doors and faucets are handy and easier to use than knobs.

If your parent or you is hoping to remain in your own home for as long as possible, ask your doctor to place an order for a "home health occupational therapy home safety evaluation" for you. This is a covered Medicare benefit, even if you are not homebound. A trained occupational therapist can assess your home and make recommendations for things to make it safer while giving you tips on which devices will make life easier for you.

All of us hope to maintain independence for as long as possible. Many of today's aids are more functional and practical to use than ever before. Aids don't represent "giving up" or "giving in." Rather, just the opposite is true. They can help your senses, your balance, and your overall quality of life as you age.

It's time to put aside the image of the little old lady with her walker. Take charge of your life by finding the best aids for you. Make them the tools for your freedom, not your frustration, so that you can continue to enjoy the people and things you love most.

· 25 ·

Delirious

"*I'*m worried about Inez," Alonzo disclosed one warm midsummer afternoon. He had driven my mother to our farm for a visit. My mom was now happily ensconced on the deck, watching the lambs and talking to Emily about her upcoming eighteenth birthday and plans for college next fall.

"What's wrong?" I asked.

"Inez's cardiologist told her she needed to rest. Her heart is growing worse."

Knowing Inez, we both were aware how impossible it was for her to slow down. "Quit fussing over me," Inez would reprimand Alonzo whenever he expressed concern. "Fuss over Margaret."

Alonzo looked uneasy. "I'm also a little concerned about your mother. She had a hard time getting up and dressed today. That's not like her, especially when she knows she's coming to your house."

Seeing her through the window fully engaged and laughing, I dismissed it as an anomaly. I was more troubled over Inez.

"Alonzo, why don't you take some time off to be with her? Mariana said she could work more hours, and for the time being, Mom is doing well."

He looked torn and said he would think about it, making me promise not to tell my mother about Inez, knowing it could upset her.

Dinner was around a campfire in the pasture, and my mother enjoyed roasting a hot dog on a stick. At eighty-nine years old, for someone who had lost so much, she always tried to retain a positive attitude and was still game for anything—like eating s'mores. She seemed tired when we took her home at nine o'clock, but she said she'd had a wonderful time and was looking forward to two days hence and coming to Emily's birthday party. The only complaint was that a small glob of melted marshmallow got stuck in her hair; we all knew she had a sensitive scalp.

"Don't touch it!" she had exclaimed as I tried pulling the sticky goo out. "Anyway, I'm having my hair done tomorrow. Tina will do it."

Alonzo greeted me with the news that Inez was feeling better, then noted the smell of campfire on our clothes and saw the sugar adhered to my mother's hair. "Your mother—she is such a good sport," he said, smiling, "like Inez."

The next morning, though, Alonzo called early. The anxiety in his voice was obvious, and I assumed it was related to Inez. It wasn't. He relayed that my mother had awakened repeatedly during the night complaining her hair was sticking to her pillow, and now she didn't want to get out of bed. She kept muttering something about "the other woman."

"After her hair appointment, let her nap today," I replied, not overly concerned, "and get her to bed early tonight."

That afternoon, however, when she phoned, her words pulled me up short.

"I don't need that cemetery plot next to Daddy anymore," she said, with uncharacteristic shakiness to her tone. "He's moving."

For an instant I wanted to laugh, then realized she was serious. "Moving? Moving where, Mom?"

"Actually, he's already moved . . . to be with that other woman. Daddy doesn't love me anymore." Her voice was on the verge of tears.

For over sixty years, the only woman in my father's life was my mother. "What are you talking about? What other woman?"

"Eleanor," she whispered, "from that place."

"You mean Eleanor from Montavilla?"

"Yes."

"Mom, you're dreaming! You didn't sleep well last night."

"Daddy wants to be buried next to her," she continued, heartbreakingly. "Not by me. He told me so."

Alonzo took the phone as my mother broke down. He explained that she had still not eaten or drunk anything today and that the hairdresser, Tina, had told him that Margaret didn't seem herself.

I placed a call to Dr. Moore. Unfortunately, he was out of town on vacation for a week, but his on-call partner returned my phone call and listened briefly to my description of my mother's symptoms. Rapidly diagnosing her symptoms as "failure to thrive," he said that the drug she was recently put on for a urinary tract infection probably hadn't had time to be effective yet. He assured me that she should be better tomorrow.

It was a weekend, and Alonzo went home to be with Inez. Mariana came over to stay the night. Saturday morning she called at 8:00 a.m., reporting that my mother was worse. She had not slept all night and now was too weak to get out of bed.

Today was Emily's eighteenth birthday. Sitting at the breakfast table with John, Emily, and Jennifer, I had to make a choice. We were planning to go hiking on Mt. Hood to celebrate, and it was a two-hour drive to the trailhead. I hated to disrupt the plans.

"You need to check on her and we'll wait to go until we hear from you," insisted John. "Hopefully, your mom is better when you get there."

"I'm sorry—"

"Don't be sorry. These things happen."

Yes they did, but they always seemed to happen at inconvenient times, I thought, and then felt guilty all over again on all counts. My mother needed me, but so did my husband and kids. Once more, I recollected the searing words an acquaintance had said to me. She had three children and much younger, involved, and *healthy* parents. Her comment was not meant to be mean spirited, merely observational. But they cut to the quick just the same:

"Your holidays seem like they're always spent at the hospital. How unfortunate. All your kids know is sick grandparents."

John easily brushed off the comment. He said Emily and Jennifer had not been ruined; moreover, they had grown into empathetic persons. Helping grandparents when they were sick was not a bad thing, he maintained.

But the guilt poured in nonetheless.

Upon reaching her home, I found my mother was in worse shape than I expected. Mariana was wringing her hands.

"When I try to give her a sip of water, she just closes her lips tight," she said, bewildered.

I brought the glass to my mom, but with her hand she pushed it aside.

"Come here," she said, motioning for me to listen without being over-heard. I leaned my ear close to her face. "She's trying to poison me," whispered my mother, frantically pointing a finger at Mariana. "She and Alonzo. They're trying to kill me!"

Astonished, I stepped back. "Mom, I think you're dehydrated. No one is trying to poison you. You need to drink."

"I am so thirsty," she said, hoarsely, her throat dry. "But the water . . . is poison."

Mariana walked over closer. Seeing her, my mother recoiled in fear, like she was afraid Mariana was going to hurt her. Mariana's large brown eyes were full of tears.

"I'm going to call an ambulance," I said, frightened. "Stay with her."

As they loaded her into the ambulance and I climbed into the front seat to accompany her, my mother told the paramedics she needed their help to "escape." When they asked what she needed to escape from, she said her family.

"They're trying to kill me," she implored again. "Please help me."

The paramedics didn't say much after that. But they surreptitiously surveyed me throughout the entire ride to the hospital.

When we reached the emergency department, a physician ordered a urine culture and blood tests for my mother. Detecting some rattling in her lungs, she also asked for a chest x-ray. Initial results revealed my mother still had a urinary tract infection as well as signs of early pneumonia. Since she had not had anything to drink for over a day, to be on the safe side, the doctor decided to admit her to the hospital where she could get IV fluids and continue with her antibiotic, Levaquin, to treat her infection.

I brought up my mother's clouded thinking about being "poisoned." The emergency room doctor had a quick answer.

"We see this all the time. Demented elderly often have hallucinations," she explained.

"But my mother doesn't have dementia. And she's never acted like this before."

"Hmmm," she said, brushing the comment aside.

The wait for a hospital room took seven hours. John, Emily, and Jennifer did not go to Mt. Hood, putting it off until another time. They all arrived in the evening to see Nana at the same time that Mariana stopped by too, somewhat harried. She offered to spend the night with my mother so that I could go home, have dinner, and celebrate Emily's birthday. She also mentioned that Alonzo would not be coming by in the morning as Inez was not feeling well.

I quickly deliberated. After spending ten hours at the hospital, I wanted to leave and spend at least a few hours with Emily. Yet my mother, while calmer and on IVs, was still addled. Mariana, though, was already settling in for the evening. I decided to go.

"All right; thank you Mariana."

Emily, sitting on Nana's bed, leaned over to say good-bye. My mother's eyes grew wide with alarm. Seeing her preparing to depart, she grabbed Emily's arm hastily. "I need to tell you something," she said. "Just you or Jennifer."

A little baffled, Emily bent down.

"Please don't go; I'm so glad you're here!" she murmured in Emily's ear. "Your mom and dad are trying to poison me!"

Emily saw tears in her grandmother's eyes and was disturbed.

"Nana, they would never do that. They love you! We all love you!"

Immediately, her grandmother dropped her hand and, pulling away with a faint cry, shut her eyes. Tears rolled onto her pillow.

"So—you, too," she muttered out loud, in desperation. "Even *you* are poisoning me."

· 26 ·

Paging Doctor HIP!

 $\mathcal{T}$ he following morning my mother was even more wound up and rattled. When I arrived, she failed to recognize me. Mariana, worn out herself, said that for a second night in a row, my mother had not slept a wink, even though they had given her a sleeping pill called "benz" something. If anything, Mariana added, the drug seemed to increase her agitation.

Upon querying the nurse about this alarming behavior, she explained it was not unusual in the elderly. She reported that doctors were ordering an ultrasound of my mother's kidney to see if it were the cause of the problem. When the results came back, though, they were negative. The problem was not her kidney.

The problem was: What was her problem?

Observing her growing worse only accelerated my unease. Once more I called Dr. Moore's office but was again told he was out of town for the rest of the week. Then, to my surprise, I was informed that the office policy had changed. As long as my mother was in the hospital, Dr. Moore would not be able to see my mother. Her care would be provided by a *hospitalist*.

I didn't understand the term.

"A hospitalist is a board-certified physician who specializes in treating patients when they are in the hospital," explained Dr. Moore's nurse. "Many medical offices are choosing to go this route now for many reasons. What this means is that Dr. Moore isn't your mother's care provider when she is in the hospital; the hospitalist is. He or she will be the one to coordinate all her care."

I hung up feeling unsettled. Who was this hospitalist, my mother's new doctor? Did this doctor know about all her conditions and the potpourri of prescriptions she took?

All day my mother remained awake, and by evening she still had not slept at all. Other than being transported for her ultrasound, she lay immobilized in her bed, hour after hour, becoming increasingly incoherent. At six, the nurse came in saying that the doctor had prescribed the sleeping pill for another night. Mariana, arriving at ten, said she hoped it would work. She blanched at the sight of my mother. After two sleepless nights, she didn't recognize either of us now.

Yet just as the previous night, the sleeping medication seemed only to rev up my mother more, said Mariana the next morning. Through the long, dreary night, my mother had sung illogical songs, rumpled her bed sheets, and made unintelligible grunting noises. Mariana appeared drained, but my mother was a total wreck. She was far worse than when entering the hospital, and three days without sleep had turned her into a lunatic. I sent Mariana home and sat down to wait, eager to speak to the hospitalist.

But no one came. At noon, a nurse stopped in, apologizing for the delay.

"It's been terribly busy here today. Someone should be by before long to see your mother."

"I hope so," I said, distressed. "Look at her!"

Still more hours dragged, and no hospitalist came in. Exasperated, I walked to the white board where all the patients in the ward were listed with their room numbers and doctors. My mother's physician was noted as Dr. HIP. So the hospitalist had a name, even if it were an odd one. With accelerating impatience, I went back to the room to wait for Dr. Hip, finding it excruciatingly difficult to look at my mother—who, with each passing hour, was becoming more like an animal than a human being.

By mid-afternoon, her erratic behavior took yet another dive; her movements were turning spasmodic. Frightened, I saw her eyes growing more open and staring, as she lay on her bed, flailing her arms and moaning.

Once more I trekked to the nurse's station to beseech someone for help. But the refrain was the same: the doctor will be coming.

Damn Dr. Hip! Where was he/she? An aide brought food to the room at 6:00 p.m., but my mother couldn't eat. She had not touched a bite of food for three days. Now her mouth was bleeding from where she had taken a chunk out of her tongue.

Seeing the blood on her pillow and sheets, I stormed for the fifth time in five hours to track down my mother's nurse. Shifts had changed, and this one was the evening provider. She had already lost patience with me.

"I keep telling you, we can't do anything more than what we're doing! Your mother is on fluids and antibiotics. The doctor has changed sleeping aids, and she'll be given it tonight at ten."

"Why not give her the sleeping pill now? She hasn't slept for three days!"

"Sorry; those are the orders."

"So when will Dr. Hip be by? I have been waiting since this morning."

The nurse regarded me strangely. "Dr. *Hip*? All the doctors are busy with patients—"

"Well, isn't my mother a patient?" I cried. Helpless, I walked back into her hospital room. I watched my mother thrashing, delusional, waving her hands in the air. Where the hell was Dr. Hip?

Suddenly I could witness such suffering no longer. Pivoting on my heel, I marched back to the nurses' station.

"Okay, how much will it take?" I said. This time the nurse didn't even bother to respond. I had become invisible. She turned her back to me.

Seething, I asked again. "How much will it take to get attention for my mother?"

Slowly, the nurse turned around, frowning. "I've already told you. The doctor will be by—"

"I know, I know," I interrupted her. "*That's* not what I'm asking. I'm asking, how much will it take for you to give my mother her sleeping pill *now*?"

"She will receive it at ten."

"You don't understand. My mother is lying in the bed in sheer misery, crying out like a wounded animal caught in a trap, and Dr. Hip hasn't been by all day."

The nurse grew huffy. "There is no such person as Dr. Hip."

"It says so—on that board!"

"HIP stands for Hospital Inpatient Providers. They're a group of hospitalists."

Right now I didn't care who saw my mother, *any* doctor would do. What was critical was she needed to sleep. "So how much will it take?" I repeated anxiously.

Squinting her eyes, the nurse glimpsed me like I was the delusional one. Perhaps I was.

"I don't know what you're talking about," she intoned flatly.

"Fifty dollars? A hundred? A thousand? Ten thousand? I'll pay it! I'll pay it if you give my mother *attention*! She's suffering! Give her the sleeping pill *now* for God's sake!"

Disgusted, the nurse stormed toward another patient's room. Undaunted, I followed her to the door.

"Please, help her," I begged. "Please don't write her off!" But she ignored me.

Not knowing where else to turn, overwhelmed with defeat, I returned to my mother's room. My cell phone was going off. Seeing it was Mariana, I answered.

"Do you want me to come in tonight?" she asked.

"No, thank you, but I'm planning on staying tonight myself. You need some rest. Alonzo will be here in the morning."

"That's why I'm calling," she replied, uneasily. "Alonzo asked me to phone you. He won't be coming to see Margaret tomorrow. He says he hopes she gets better."

She paused for an instant before continuing. "He wanted me to tell you he doesn't know when he'll be back. You see, Inez just had a heart attack."

What Delirium Is and Why It's Essential You Know How to Spot It

ELIZABETH ECKSTROM, MD, MPH, MACP

$\mathcal{D}$elirium is a medical emergency that can lead to permanent cognitive impairment if not treated early and accurately. Unfortunately, it is too often unrecognized by doctors and nurses, resulting in suffering, like Marcy's mom, or even death that, if the delirium had been caught earlier, could have been prevented.

The symptoms of delirium are intense and often happen quickly. People with delirium may have personality changes, exhibiting paranoia, extreme anxiety, uncharacteristic irritability, and even combativeness. They have waxing and waning mental status; one minute they seem fine and the next, completely illogical. They usually cannot remember things and will often act very strangely to others. As many as half of older people who are hospitalized develop delirium, and for those who do, the hospital death rate can be over 50 percent. Even if someone with delirium survives a hospitalization, up to 40 percent of people who had delirium die within a year.

These are scary statistics. Even worse, they are often avoidable. If the correct cause (or causes) of delirium is recognized and addressed, the patient will recover with the least possible brain damage.

Sixty percent of physicians miss diagnosing inpatient delirium. How can that be? Why do hospitals and doctors and emergency room providers and nurses often fail to recognize delirium? The paramount reason is that most healthcare providers have not been trained to recognize delirium for what it is and how it manifests in people over sixty-five.

In too many cases, delirium is often incorrectly diagnosed as *dementia*. Rather than recognizing that a patient is acting abnormally, the doctor assumes this is the patient's baseline and fails to initiate a workup for delirium. When this happens, consequences for an elderly patient can be disastrous.

Delirium results from a variety of sources and often is due to multiple factors. This means that figuring out which factors are precipitating the delirium can be problematic. In the elderly, delirium can be triggered by infections, such as urinary tract infections, metabolic problems such as high blood sugar, lack of sleep, trauma, surgery, pain, alcohol withdrawal, and even side effects from certain drugs commonly prescribed for older adults.

It can also be caused from the hospitalization experience itself. If older patients are not given frequent orientation as to where they are when they are in the hospital, or if they are immobilized or even kept from sleeping by being awakened all night long for tests, delirium can result.

If the causes of delirium are not determined rapidly, the patient may receive the completely wrong treatment for the delirium. When this happens and delirium continues to mount, one out of two hospitalized patients will die.

What are the symptoms of delirium, and how can it be differentiated from dementia, which is not a medical emergency? Delirium has five cardinal features that any caregiver or family member should be aware of and seek medical attention for immediately if apparent:

1. *Rapid onset of uncharacteristic behaviors.* This is the most important indicator of delirium. Unlike dementia, which is a progressive cognitive decline that happens gradually over months or years, delirium symptoms appear abruptly, usually in days or even hours.

2. *Dramatic symptoms and profoundly altered mental status.* Delirium behaviors are different from a person's normal performance. This is a powerful clue. Many people with delirium experience hallucinations, delusions, and paranoia—which can be terrifying to the patient and very distressing for a family member or hospital staff to experience. A person with delirium can express feeling threatened by bizarre and irrational things—like a shadow on the wall or imagining snakes are in the room.

3. *Disorganized thinking.* Older patients with delirium cannot focus. Often their speech is incoherent. They may ramble on with irrelevant conversation or with an illogical flow of ideas. They may switch from subject to subject with no reasoning.

4. *Fluctuating wake/sleep patterns.* Delirious patients can alternate between being hyperactive with episodes of being extremely sleepy.

5. *Significant inattention.* Patients with delirium cannot keep track of what is being said or follow a dialogue.

Once delirium is recognized, the cause of the delirium should be found as soon as possible and corrected. In addition, the risk of developing delirium in the hospital can be reduced by the following strategies, all of which should be a part of an older person's hospital care plan:

1. *Frequent orientation.* Family members and hospital staff need to regularly remind patients why they are in the hospital, what day it is, and other points of reference to help patients keep track of their surroundings.

2. *Reduce sensory problems.* If patients depend on aids to see or hear, it is critical that hearing aids and glasses are always on during the hospital stay. This ensures that they can keep up with their medical issues and recognize the many people who come in to care for them.

3. *Maintain adequate hydration.* When confused by being in the hospital, many older persons don't drink well. Medical illnesses like infections can also lead to dehydration. Family and staff need to be attentive and help older patients drink enough fluids.

4. *Manage sleep.* Older people often sleep poorly in the hospital; this in itself can increase the risk of developing delirium. Sleeping pills for people over sixty-five can be unsafe and have dangerous side effects. It is much better to use gentle music, a back rub, warm milk or herbal tea, and other non-drug strategies to help improve sleep.

5. *Keep active during the day.* Even when in the hospital, patients need to be up and doing things during the day whenever possible. It is beneficial if they eat in their chair rather than the bed, avoid watching TV, and walk or exercise. Being active helps to lessen sleep disturbances and reduce the onset of delirium.

6. *Treat pain adequately.* Too much pain or too many pain pills can both cause delirium. It is therefore imperative to monitor a patient closely to determine the right amount of medication to alleviate pain without causing side effects. This is not easy and is even harder if someone has dementia and is not able to accurately report his or her pain levels.

Although the two are often confused, delirium is *not* dementia. Whereas dementia is irreversible and progressive, delirium is not. Delirium is a life-threatening emergency that has a rapid onset. If its underlying causes are swiftly and adequately treated, brain damage often is not permanent. But this requires family members and friends to clearly communicate with the hospital team when they notice unusual behavior and the hospital team to work diligently to prevent and treat delirium.

Like Marcy, if you suspect your parent is exhibiting delirium, don't wait. Get your parent to the hospital. And if the hospital provider does not understand the difference between delirium and dementia nor seeks to find the underlying causes of the rapid change in behavior, don't give up until you find a provider who does. A good team—doctor, nurse, social worker, pharmacist, and therapist—working together and with involved family members can provide optimal prevention and treatment of delirium. How soon it is recognized and managed can affect its outcome . . . and make all the difference between life and death.

"Sometimes It's Better
If They Never Wake Up"

*J*ust before ten o'clock, my mother finally collapsed. I wasn't sure whether to be relieved or even more frightened. Her sleep was so deep, it seemed like a coma. Two hours later, a doctor at last showed up and stood in the room's doorway. He commented that he was not her provider but had been summoned. Seeing her asleep, he said he would not bother to examine her. Her doctor would be by in the morning.

To my bewilderment, he then faced me and crossed his arms.

"This is what Pope John Paul died of, you know. An infected bladder. If she comes out of this, you can expect a real step down in her functioning. That's been my experience. She's what? Eighty-five, ninety years old?"

I was stunned to silence.

"At times like these," he advised gently, "sometimes it's better if they never wake up."

But my mother was still alive in the morning when the real "Dr. Hip" made rounds to see her. Hip was not his actual name, of course. In fact, I came to understand there were two or three hospitalists who rotated, taking turns in caring for my mother. None had known her before, and we had had no relationship. I found it easier just to think of them all as "Dr. Hip."

After only one interaction with Dr. Hip Number One—who was to be the main doctor we dealt with—I found myself lamenting for the time when one's primary care doctor still saw his or her own patients in the hospital. Dr. Moore's compassion and holistic understanding of my mother's composite of problems were not in evidence in the thirty-five-year-oldish man with the crew cut and wire-rimmed glasses who examined my mother. Belying his tony name, Dr. Hip was all business. And while I appreciated the fact that he took the time to listen to her heart and lungs and review her recent lab work, he seemed unable to comprehend that my mother was not *like* this just four days ago. Nothing I could do or say seemed to change his concept of her as just another sick old lady.

"Your mother still has a UTI—urinary tract infection—and I am going to change her antibiotic. Levaquin doesn't appear to be effective."

"How long until she comes out of this?"

Dr. Hip was writing something in the chart. "Out of what?"

"This paranoia." It was the thing that worried me the most. "The terrible hallucinations."

"In a person with dementia," he replied, "it's difficult to tell."

"But my mother doesn't have dementia." It was the third time I had told a medical professional the same thing. Why did it seem to make no impact at all?

"Healthy brains don't respond to infections in this way. It's a product of her baseline dementia," corrected Dr. Hip.

"This isn't normal for her; she's had infections before."

But Dr. Hip had stuffed the chart back in the box and was on his way out. So what was I doing wrong? Was I speaking a foreign language?

"You are going to be okay," I patted my mother, who lay in her bed unspeaking, her mouth agape with saliva collecting in its corner. Right now she looked every day of her eighty-nine years old . . . and demented.

Dr. Hip ordered a PICC line, or catheter, to be implanted in my mother's arm and chest to administer the new antibiotic. Unfortunately, after it was inserted, it seemed to continually clog. By evening, it seemed we had traded one serious problem for another.

As a reaction to the rounds of fluids given to flush out the blocked line, my mother developed a wheeziness to her breathing. She would wake up gasping for air and then fall back to sleep again, exhausted. Nurses came in to nebulize her—a procedure common to open airways for asthmatics—but her respirations continued to be labored.

Dr. Hip called the new condition "congestive heart failure," which I knew something about. My mother's cardiologist had previously diagnosed her with a mild case, but now, plied with all the extra fluids being poured into her to rectify a stubborn PICC line, my mother's symptoms had become much more pronounced. Two of the most notable warning signals were swollen ankles and legs and, of greater concern, as lungs began filling with fluid, difficulty breathing. Both were in evidence.

To try to "dehydrate" her, Dr. Hip put her on a dose of Lasix. I asked the nurse whether the hospitalist knew that my mother had her own cardiologist who would probably want to know about this new "turn" in her congestive heart failure.

The nurse shook her head. "Probably not."

"Do you think I should call the cardiologist?"

"If she were my mother, I would," said the nurse. "But it's up to you."

I made the call. The cardiologist said she would contact Dr. Hip to discuss my mother's health history. I felt somewhat relieved, that is, until the next time I met with Dr. Hip, when he admonished me that I had interfered with protocol.

"It is not your prerogative to call in a specialist," exhorted Dr. Hip. "You must understand, when your mother is here, in this hospital, *I* make the decisions. I would ask you to please refrain from interfering."

Elizabeth Ross happened to be visiting during Dr. Hip's rounds and overheard my chastisement. Her shoulders stiffened.

"I discuss cases with specialists when I deem it necessary," he continued. "In fact, I had lunch today with two infectious disease experts and brought up your mother's stubborn UTI and history of infections. These doctors said they would not even bother to treat her, at her age. But I have decided to do it anyway," he said, grandly.

"Well, isn't that just peachy," said Elizabeth, after he left. She was livid. "It's probably against his better judgment, though. My God, Marcy! What he's really saying is the best course would be to just let your mother go septic and die! What if you weren't here? What do old people do that don't have advocates?"

Alonzo, calling to give me updates on Inez, said he wished he could be in two places at once. He would gladly advocate for both Inez and Margaret. In fact, Inez was concerned more for my mother than for herself, which was typical of her.

She was still in the hospital, stable for the time being, but surgery was being considered. To me, Inez seemed to have no shortage of advocates. Alonzo said a host of relatives—sometimes as many as thirty-two—were flooding the hospital to take turns being with her every moment.

"In El Salvadoran culture, when someone gets sick, we all draw together to stay with them," Alonzo explained. "Inez's doctor knows that. She's learned to just put up with all the visitors. It's not that way in America. I feel sorry for your mother. Without you, John, and your girls, she is all alone. Your sisters live far away. That is one thing our people have—lots of family. But remember," he added, in an effort to cheer me up, "Margaret is like family to us. If we weren't here, we would be with you."

Doped up on drugs, my mother floated in and out of reality for several days. The good news was that the fluid in her lungs was reducing with the Lasix therapy, thanks, to be fair, to Dr. Hip. But there was bad news. Her respirations remained shallow, which predisposed her to worsening pneumonia.

Dr. Hip called a respiratory therapist on board to administer albuterol and oxygen nebulizers several times a day. For two days, the therapy seemed to improve her overall wheeziness, which I found encouraging. But then, one morning, the nebulizing abruptly stopped.

I questioned the nurse and learned that Dr. Hip had arranged it. He had also given a subsequent order: to halt all further treatment.

On his morning rounds, the doctor explained his reasoning.

"Respiratory therapy is doing no good for your mother. It does not work in cases of aspiration pneumonia. Actually, your mother should have been discharged from here three days ago. There is nothing more we can do for her."

"So you're sending her home?" I asked.

"No, I'm sending her to a convalescent center where she can continue with her antibiotics for a while longer. But understand, there is a haziness on the x-ray of her right lung, most likely due to aspiration."

"What's that mean?"

"Demented elderly will aspirate on just about anything, even their own saliva. In these cases, antibiotics aren't helpful and tube feedings do no good."

My head was beginning to spin. "So what does that mean?"

"It means there is no cure."

A sudden weakness traveled down my arms, and I worked to steady myself. "Wait a minute; I don't get it. How can dementia happen this fast? Just a week ago my mother was roasting hotdogs around a campfire! She was laughing, talking, and with it. How can someone go so quickly from normal to being in the end stage of aspiration pneumonia? You said yourself, she has an infection!"

"Let me put it another way," said Dr. Hip, growing a little impatient with my lack of comprehension. "To exhibit the kind of irrationality that your mother has displayed ever since entering the hospital, a patient would have to have underlying dementia. Yesterday you told me about your father's history of Alzheimer's. He probably died of aspiration pneumonia from his own saliva."

"That's not so!" I exclaimed. "He caught viral pneumonia from the nursing home! And my mother doesn't have Alzheimer's!"

"Demented people eventually aspirate. That's the way it is. There is nothing more I can do for your mother," said Dr. Hip decisively.

The brutal significance of his speech took over my emotions. I panicked. What could I say to make him *listen*? Yesterday the respiratory therapist said that the nebulizing was helping my mother. Now Dr. Hip had halted it for good. Frantically, I thought of my father. Even if the news had been bad, he would never have broken it like this. He was a healer; he had compassion.

There was nothing healing or compassionate about Dr. Hip.

"Since she will be leaving later today, there'll be some forms for you to sign," he said, continuing to rattle off more instructions, including something about my "choice" for "final facilities." But I couldn't follow the words. My thoughts lagged behind my shock. All I heard was Dr. Hip saying my mother was being sent to a nursing home—to die.

"I don't believe you!" I interrupted. "My mother is not dying!"

Dr. Hip didn't respond to my outburst; to him I was merely acting hysterical. "I can't really tell you anything more," he said, professionally. "I'd advise you to accept the inevitable. After all, you saw your father's course."

What I Wish I'd Known

The Most Important Medical Word That Can Save Your Parent's Life—"Baseline"

ELIZABETH ECKSTROM, MD, MPH, MACP

*O*lder persons enter the hospital with myriad presenting reasons: urinary tract infections, pneumonias, influenza, trauma from falls, congestive heart failure, or many other problems. One important thing that should be on every family member's mind when an elderly loved one arrives at an emergency room, is to make sure that the care provider understands the patient's *baseline*. Too often, this vital piece of information is overlooked. This simple bit of "doctor-speak" can make all the difference in an elderly patient's outcome—whether the patient ends up going home, to a nursing home, or, in some cases, never making it out of the hospital.

Baseline is a patient's *normal* functioning level and should cover both physical and cognitive function. For physical function, it is best to consider "activities of daily living," such as: is the patient presently living independently and taking care of herself? If not, what is she able to do herself? What does she need help to perform, such as bathing and taking medication? When describing people's baseline, it is also important to include their current mental status. Do they have trouble with their memory or with managing complex tasks like doing finances? Have they been diagnosed with dementia? The more a family member can be specific about these *baseline* characteristics for the health team, the better job that team will be able to do caring for the patient.

Doctors and healthcare providers need this knowledge to help accurately diagnose and treat the patient's problems. Too often, when an old person comes to the hospital exhibiting any kind of confusion, the symptoms are treated as the patient's *baseline* because the person is old and unfamiliar to the care team. This can lead to underappreciation of a new *decline* in cognition or physical function.

This is where the family can come in. When a patient is not acting like himself or herself, family members can offer invaluable information on a patient's pertinent health history. Unfortunately, in a busy hospital setting, there is often not a lot of time for discussion. Some issues that may be important and shed light on the current situation could be overlooked. For this reason, you can do two valuable things before a crisis arises that can help speed up proper and critical treatment for your parent.

First, understand what your parent's *current baseline* is. Ask his or her primary doctor for a quick, written assessment or to review an appraisal that you have written. This needn't be longer than one paragraph but should include your parent's present physical and mental level of function (for example, "Dad can normally walk about ten blocks, does most of the cooking for himself and Mom, and never forgets to take his pills or get to an appointment on time.")

Second, create a *health history sheet* for your parent. This can be one page and should be reviewed by your parent's doctor for accuracy. It should include your parent's name, date of document, date of birth, insurance carrier, primary care doctor and phone, primary contact person and phone, and current address. It should also list who has your parent's power of attorney.

It should list all medications your parent is on, the current dosage, and what each medication is taken for. These can be divided into groups: morning, afternoon, evening, and bedtime medications.

It should list any allergies to medications and any special needs your parent might have (hearing aids, walker, etc.).

The final paragraph(s) should be a summary of your parent's medical history. These would include her present *baseline status*, for example, "alert, oriented, and cooperative, with little or no memory trouble," and major medical conditions, such as "congestive heart failure," "atrial fibrillation," and "orthostatic hypotension." Included here would be a short history of prior hospitalizations.

If your parent has completed advance directives and/or a POLST, document that on the health history sheet as well.

For an excellent example of a health history sheet, and a template you can use, see Appendix 2.

This health history sheet provides vital information quickly to your parent's doctor or hospitalist. It can be printed on a regular-sized piece of typing/printer paper—bright colors are unmistakable—and laminated and kept on your parent's refrigerator or near the front door so that you won't forget about it in an emergency. One can be kept in your parent's purse or wallet, and every caregiver and family member should have a copy. In this way, a person's health status and needs are up-to-date and easily retrievable. It will be available for paramedics to review should the need arise and will help the doctor in any emergency situation have a clearer picture of the older person's healthcare issues, which can be extremely beneficial.

While the health history sheet will provide valuable information for the health team, family members can also be extremely helpful adjuncts to the care team of doctors, nurses, pharmacists, and therapists. Perhaps more than anyone else, family members can help in recognizing fluctuating mental status, inattention, and other key delirium features. They can also be vital members of the patient's treatment plan, helping to implement activity and other programs to reduce the dangerous but common illness, delirium.

In Marcy's case, if she had only known the "magic" words *"This is not my mother's baseline,"* and produced a health history sheet to *certify it*, it may have prevented many days of unintended anguish for her mother and alleviated her own despair.

· 28 ·

Where Old People Are Sent to Die

$\mathcal{U}$nable to breathe, I leaned against the door as the world whirled around me.

"Are you all right?" asked a nurse, placing her hand on my shoulder. I recognized her as the kind attendant who had looked after my mother for the past three days.

I nodded as the tears fell down my cheeks. I needed to call John. I needed his support, and I needed it right away.

"We all want your mother to be comfortable," she said gently. "I'm sure you want that too."

My reply, I knew, should have been "Of course," but my heart wouldn't let me say it. Rather, what rose up was the one question that had been demanding utterance.

"Would my mother be given this kind of treatment if she were fifty, not ninety?"

A troubled expression crossed the nurse's face, like she didn't know how to respond. Taking a moment to answer, she lowered her voice.

"No."

"I know," I whispered.

"The West Ridge"—"*A Compassionate Care Facility*"—was one of the nicer nursing homes in the city. Before my mother arrived in her private room, I was given a tour of the facility's services—the dining room, the TV center, the activities room—all the amenities my mother presumably would not be needing, considering she was demented and dying of aspiration pneumonia, according to Dr. Hip.

Admittedly, unlike the other critical care centers I had experienced, this one was actually attractive. It had windows facing flowered courtyards, pleasant seating areas with comfortable chairs, and even a highly varnished grand piano that continually played restful music in the lobby. The piano, while beautiful to gaze upon, was also kind of creepy—it performed on and on automatically—like fingers of ghosts running up and down the keys.

But farther down the corridors, the hallmark aroma of wet Depends became evident. Instinctually, that odor still gave me the fight-or-flight response. Houses didn't smell like that, nor did hospitals. It struck me that if a nursing home didn't have that lingering scent, visitors might possibly come more often and stay longer.

I waited for my "care conference" by a plastic poinsettia plant, which seemed a little early to put out, considering Christmas was still five months away. When the receptionist informed me they were ready, I was led into a long, narrow room where an assemblage of providers sat around a conference table. The "team" consisted of a social worker, head nurse, physical therapist, and occupational therapist all brought together to discuss my mother's "care plan." Right away I got the feeling that everyone considered it a perfunctory obligation—more like a pre-funeral gathering.

The professionals assured me that my mother would be kept relaxed and pain free. She was to continue on IV antibiotics for one more week. At least, I thought, Dr. Hip had conceded that, even if his caveat was that they wouldn't do any good. Every face in the room had the "it's just a matter of time" look that was becoming achingly familiar. When I professed that my mother never had dementia before this, their expressions became even more fixedly pessimistic. Only one, the charge nurse, Alice, did not seem entirely in lockstep with the death sentence. "It's really up to your mother now," she said, at the meeting's conclusion.

"What did you mean when you said that—that it was up to my mom?" I asked her as we exited.

"We get lots of patients from the hospital. Some come from HIP. They're all good doctors, but sometimes they're wrong. Sometimes the patients don't die. They just get sent here to do so.

"On the other hand," she retracted quickly, like throwing a lifeline she hadn't meant to, "I've seen too many times where families pull out all the stops but the patient doesn't want them to. The patient just wants to be let go. I think the most important thing is what are the *patient's wishes.*"

With a significant glance, Alice returned to her job of dispensing a rolling table full of medicine vials. Lights down the hallway were lit, indicating patients were paging her. Similar to the other two nursing homes I knew, there never seemed to be many aides moving about, attending to all the call buttons.

John left work to help me get my mother settled in her room. I called my sisters to break the news. They would make plans to fly out in the next few days. Mariana arrived, saying she could stay nights in my mother's room; there was a chair that could be made into a bed. But the whole thing seemed wrong, somehow.

Emily and Jennifer agreed. "No one is giving Nana a chance to live," argued Jennifer. "They're all siding with Dr. Hip. How do you even know he's right?"

My sisters, when they arrived, though, were despondent. Seeing our mother hooked up to IVs and barely responsive, they believed that her time had come. While we never saw a doctor again, Alice stopped in to check on my mother several times during her shifts.

"Unless there's a real change, she's got just two more days of IV vancomycin," she informed me. "Has your mom responded at all?"

I shook my head. "Not really. She just—sleeps, and never really wakes up."

"I think it's time you may have to begin facing the facts," she replied. "I think your sisters have."

But what Alice didn't understand was that my sisters didn't live here. They hadn't seen our mother just two weeks before, laughing and eating s'mores around the campfire and talking to Emily about her birthday and college and Jennifer about following her dream of becoming a veterinarian. Did life really turn on and off like that? My father had had pneumonia; I had been there through his last week and had seen what the disease did. While Dr. Hip said this was the same thing, it sure didn't look like it.

Alice saw the conflict on my face. "I think she is waiting for you to say it's okay for her to go," she added, gently.

My sisters agreed, saying I needed to release her.

The following afternoon, with only one day remaining of antibiotics, I sat by my mother's bedside, thinking. Emily, Jennifer, and John were working, my sisters out buying groceries. My mother and I were alone in the room. It was the perfect time to free her. She *was* tired, wasn't she? She had aspiration pneumonia, didn't she? I didn't want her to suffer like she had in the hospital ever again. Aspirating on one's saliva made for those terrible hallucinations. And there was no cure. I needed to tell her it was all right to go.

"I don't know if you can hear me or not, Mom," I said to the limp figure who still had not spoken since collapsing at the hospital ten days ago. I picked up her weak hand and held it. "Everyone thinks you are going to die."

I started to cry, silently, and opened my mouth to say the final words. They caught in my throat. What came out was entirely different.

"Well, I don't."

My avowal surprised even me. But once I began, I couldn't stop.

"I *don't*! What's more, I don't want you to die! I don't believe damn Dr. Hip that you're choking to death. I don't believe you are demented. I think you're just really, really sick!"

I was doing it all wrong and I knew it, and my sisters and the nurse and everyone would be furious with me. But I didn't care.

"If what you really want is to rest, fine. I'll try to accept that. But, Mom, if you want me to fight for you, I'll fight!"

With every bit of my heart reaching into her heart, I laid my head on her arm. "You've got to let me know what you want! *Do you want to live?*"

The faint squeeze on my hand said it all.

The Lazarus Syndrome

$\mathcal{B}$ursting into the hall, I hunted the corridors until I tracked down Alice.

"She wants to live," I said. "She needs to continue with her IV antibiotic."

The nurse stared at me skeptically. "The orders are to discontinue it tomorrow."

"Well, we've got to change that."

"That's difficult . . ."

"So what do we do?"

"Nothing; we don't change anything . . . unless there is real improvement," she replied, unconvinced.

"There is real improvement," I said emphatically. "She wants to live. She has a history of beating the odds. Give her a chance."

It was true; throughout my mother's life, there seemed to be numerous times when she just squeaked by. She had escaped death's clutches by a twist of fate, quick thinking, or, like my father, not panicking in a situation. Several episodes rose up in my mind . . .

When she was six years old, she had missed death when she fell off the bridge at Multnomah Falls and was caught only by her father's swift reflexes.

She had narrowly missed it years later when, at the last moment, she decided not to go riding in the car with her parents the night they were hit head-on and killed.

She evaded it yet again when the small powerboat in which she was riding unexpectedly had a gas leak and exploded. She had just gotten up from the chair she was sitting in when it blew up and was thrown into the water. Then the entire craft caught fire and sank. She survived.

She had sidestepped it once more when their plane was forced to land on the Texas freeway.

And she had potentially thwarted it the fateful day my father had borrowed a friend's floatplane for a pleasure flight up the Columbia Gorge. Perhaps that time was not really death defying. But it still had been terrifying, just the same . . .

My mother hadn't yet learned how to fly, and she was not wild over floatplanes. My dad, though, entreated that she would love the experience—the feeling of arising from the river, flying by Mount Hood and the Cascades, and landing again on the blue Columbia. Part of the fun, he'd said, was that the little plane was a single-prop that needed a manual push to get going.

With my mother in the copilot seat, my father stood on the pontoon to give a heave to the propeller. They were already freed of the dock and floating rather rapidly down the swift Columbia. For the first two tries, the motor didn't start.

"Don't fall in!" yelled my mother, seeing him balance unsteadily as waves chopped at the plane. As the wind was blowing into the cockpit, she shut the door just as the third thrust jettisoned the propeller to life. My father, holding on for balance, hastened back to the door. Grasping the latch, he pulled. But it didn't move.

"Open the door!" he yelled.

Immediately she unbuckled her seatbelt and leaned over to push the door free, but the lever appeared stuck.

"Open the door!" he shouted again. With a sickening sensation, she realized the door had somehow become locked. My father's yanking did no good, and she saw him point down at something she couldn't see. A lock? She put her ear against the window.

"*Steer!*" my father was bellowing.

Directly ahead, she observed a large floating log. The plane, amassing speed in the current, was set on a crash course. Scanning the dashboard for something to steer, she could not find a wheel. My father pounded at the window; he was motioning to her feet.

Glancing down, my mother saw what looked to be pedals. Tentatively pressing one, the plane lurched to the left, nearly thrusting my dad off the pontoon. As she rapidly pushed the other, the plane changed direction and straightened. Using both pedals in tandem, my mother successfully avoided hitting the snag just in the nick of time.

My father continued hammering at the door, and she turned her attention back to the window. The small plane bounced over the waves, making it difficult to see straight as it collected speed. For a horrible second, she wondered, was it going to take off?

"Don't give in to panic," she steadied herself. "Don't give up; George is still holding on. You can *do* this . . . and kill him later."

With one eye glued to the river rushing by, the other scanning the door, and both feet steering, my mother reached to pull every knob she could see. It was then she noticed one small nubbin, stuck down beneath the windowsill. Frantically working it with her thumb and forefinger, she saw it suddenly pop back up, releasing the latch. Immediately, the door flew wide with such force it almost toppled my father backward into the river.

Catching the door frame, he managed to hoist himself into the plane. Slamming the door behind him, he fell into my mother's lap. Without a word, he maneuvered himself into the cockpit, fastened his seatbelt, and accelerated the motor. The plane, responding, rose up into the air and began gliding smoothly down the Gorge.

"Isn't this fun?" said my father at last.

"No," my mother said. "Not fun."

"You're a great girl," he remarked, with genuine admiration. "I can always count on you in an emergency to never give up."

Once more this great girl was not giving up. I wouldn't, either.

Alice stared at my determined face and relented. "All right, I'll tell the doctor there's been a change," she said, shaking her head.

The turnabout did not happen immediately, and my sisters, who had to leave for home, were uncertain my mother was on the right course. But by the week's end she had so improved that she was sitting up in her bed, eating, and talking again. By the end of the second week of the right antibiotic, her lung sounds were back to normal, and all signs of hallucinations and paranoid behaviors had passed.

"You need to send a video of Nana to Dr. Hip," said Jennifer and Emily, still upset at his treatment of their grandmother. "Show him she didn't die."

No, Dr. Hip would not believe this was the same woman he had pronounced demented and nearly DOA—dead on arrival. Alice, having been through situations like this before, later put it this way:

"There are some patients, like your mother, that we see who come back to life. With the right management, a certain amount of their own spunk, and usually some family advocacy, they seem to rise from the dead. We call it "*the Lazarus syndrome.*"

Alice was pleased by the progress; my entire family, of course, felt elated. Alonzo, visiting with Inez, who was now out of the hospital herself, spoke for all of us when he proclaimed, "Once more, Margaret, you showed all of them!"

By the third week, with Elizabeth Ross's help, my mother was up and being retrained to walk. Everyone was now encouraged—even Dr. Moore, who was her provider again now that she was out of the hospital. He said at the conclusion of her antibiotic therapy—still a couple of weeks away—he felt she should be well enough to go home. She would need some additional care, though, as she continued regaining strength. In the meantime, I cleaned her refrigerator and prepared her house in anticipation of her return.

"Please take me off your speed dial," said Alice to me one afternoon when I came to visit, bringing my mom an armload of new books on tape. "I appreciate that you're here every day, and it's great that you have Alonzo to watch your mom. We both know this place is understaffed. But now your mom is on a road to recovery. While I don't mind you calling me, you really do overdo it sometimes. I like you, but you're what we term '*high mainte-nance.*'"

I had to agree. It had been a difficult few months. For now, though, we had dodged another bullet, and that was reason to rejoice. For now, everyone was doing better and feeling better . . . managing their health and lives and activities better . . .

Everyone except me.

• 30 •

A Hope and a Future

$\mathcal{L}$ike a seesaw in motion, I reached my nadir at the same time my mother rose in her health prognosis. The crisis was past. She went up; I went down. The pieces in her life were fitting back together. Mine were falling apart.

For two months I'd been battling headaches daily. My "techniques" to try to take care of myself as well as my family were not working. I was still exercising a lot . . . running . . . running like a madwoman . . . and praying and trying to write (failing), talking with friends, "letting down" with my family, and reading "self-help" books and "caregiving" books and all the rest. They were all good practices, but right now, none of them really helped. Inside, I was tired. Inside, I felt at my wit's end. What I really wanted to say to the whole world but couldn't because the world didn't care, was:

This is all so sad!

I was discovering that when life squeezed you with pain and the person who was making you sad was still *alive*, you didn't have the time or sanction to grieve. Why? Because there was too much grinding work still to be done. There were family responsibilities, work responsibilities, caregiving responsibilities. Time was fractured, but it continued to have its demands just the same. It did not let up; it did not allow you to get off the treadmill.

In the rare, quiet moments, I knew what was wrong. It wasn't just that time was fractured. It was my heart that was broken. What was it screaming? *It hurts like hell to see this decline in the people I love the most in the world . . . my family!*

For nibble by nibble, inch by inch, before my eyes they were wearing away. I had had practice "pretending away" Alzheimer's. It wasn't successful. No matter what I did, my father still suffered that wrenching decline; now it was my mother. At times—when I would allow myself to feel—I felt caught in a vise: exhausted, hopeless. It seemed that to love so deeply in this life was to hurt so deeply!

And then, when I had a moment to stand back from caregiving, I worried: Just what sort of person was I becoming? What kind of mother was I these days? When she recovered her speech, my mother said, in appreciation but cognizant of change, "I think of *you* as my mother now." But what about my own children? How did they feel?

And John? What kind of wife was I? One too often in tears, constantly needing support or continually battling hospital administrators? One who didn't have time to cook dinners or hear about *his* day? John's patience was extraordinary. What was wrong with my patience? Why could I not handle stress? Did I have no capacity?

What about my friends? The only subject I seemed to be able to converse about was the *newest* emergency, or the *latest* fall, or still another family *crisis*. Another thing I was learning: if people hadn't gone through the devastation of Alzheimer's, they sure didn't want to hear about it. So, on top of everything else, I was turning into a lousy friend as well.

"You need to see a doctor yourself," said John one evening.

"But there's nothing wrong with me."

"Your headaches. You're having them every day."

"I'm fine," I responded. "And my mom's better. I'm taking her in to Dr. Moore next week."

"I'm not talking about your mother or her appointments," said John, concerned. "It's about *you*."

Reluctantly, I made the appointment. And as soon as I did, I regretted it.

It was humiliating to be sitting in Dr. Moore's examining room, taking up his valuable time to talk about something so minor as headaches. Everyone got headaches now and then. Everyone got tired and discouraged; I was just being a baby. If not for John, I would never have come in.

I knew exactly what I needed to do without any advice from a doctor. What I needed was to just suck it up and get on with life. In every life some rain must fall, or however the saying went. This was a case of feeling sorry for myself and exaggerating my symptoms. I should be discussing with him my *mother*, her problems. She had nearly died. We needed to talk about that. That was important. Headaches weren't. And probably, the reason behind a spate of headaches was simply a lack of sleep.

So what must Dr. Moore think of me?

My head started to throb even more just contemplating how silly I was being. It was all a waste of time. I knew busy doctors only had fifteen minutes to give to a patient. Well, I would make it easy for Dr. Moore; I would graciously take only five. I would say my headaches were improving; John and I had merely overreacted; I would consciously eat better and continue running and exercising and try to get to church now and again and feel grateful for my family and that my mother had lived and then thank Dr. Moore for his time and leave him with an extra few minutes for his next patient.

But when Dr. Moore came in, my plan didn't work out that way. After opening the door and saying hello, he sat down in the chair next to mine. He did not refer to my chart or roll over to the computer placed in the room. Rather, what he did next startled me.

He took my hand.

My first impulse was to pull away, but Dr. Moore's blue eyes were so kind that I didn't. For a moment he didn't speak but looked at my face.

"You don't have a brain tumor," he said, then added softly, "How many times did your father and mother nearly die now?"

"What do you mean?"

"I remember incidents about your father at the nursing home. I remember you telling me about his broken hip; his lack of water. Your mother, as my patient, I know has nearly passed away several times."

I wasn't sure what he was getting at, but Dr. Moore sat back in his swivel chair, not letting go of my hand. "Do you know who else suffers when a person nearly dies and then recovers, or when a loved one is poised on the fine line between life and death?" he asked.

I shook my head.

"The people who love them. And it is especially hard if one of those people is the person's caregiver. You've heard of posttraumatic stress syndrome?"

"That's what soldiers get when they return from war."

"The symptoms you have, from fighting this battle for life for your parents, not just once but numerous times, are the same. Luckily, I don't think in your case they will be as long lasting, but they are real, regardless."

He released my hand. I thought about his words. I knew I had been under stress, but I always considered that if I couldn't handle it, it was my own fault. It was my own weakness. But Dr. Moore was validating that my symptoms were real. They were not only valid, but to be expected.

"Caregivers, such as you, face tremendous pressures," he continued. "You have taken care of both of your parents for over ten years. It is a worthy and demanding job description. You have been your parents' nurse, doctor, administrator, counselor, case manager, money manager, property manager, general overseer, shopper, and everything else. There are two things you should know."

I saw from the clock on the wall that my appointment was nearing fifteen minutes. My time was up. Dr. Moore, though, did not seem to notice.

Rather, he began talking more about headaches, strain, the health of my mother, my family, John, Emily, and Jennifer, and even my writing career before coming back to his two points.

"The most critical thing of all is that you need to find more help," he said, leaning forward. "That is nothing to be ashamed of. What you need is to seek help for your mother's physical needs so that you can spend the time you have left with her concentrating on her emotional needs."

Physical needs . . . emotional needs . . . Dr. Moore was dividing them up. He was giving them equal importance in a way I had never before considered.

"That's what she really wants," he went on. "And here is the crux of the matter. If your desire is to enhance her quality of life, *you* need to have the freedom to really be with her. You, as the person who loves her, can bring her spiritual comfort. But you can't do that if you are spending every minute just tending to her physical requirements. There's not enough of you to go around."

Dr. Moore took up my hand again. His voice was calm but authoritative. "Secondly, you need to understand something about yourself. You are strong. You will get through this."

I was not expecting this . . . certainly not when I had come in complaining about a medical symptom. Dr. Moore wasn't talking about headaches, blood pressure, or cholesterol. His words reached out to touch my wounds like a healing salve.

"You are a writer. I believe someday you will write stories about your family. Write down these stories about your mother. Other people need to hear them—for you are not alone. Other people everywhere are going through the same things as you."

Something in Dr. Moore's tone filled my doubts with renewed courage. Could there really be a life caregiving? Could there be . . . a future?

"This time that you are going through is hard; you have lost your confidence," continued Dr. Moore. "But you are doing the right thing in caring for your family. And if you don't become a writer, then I think you should consider becoming a doctor."

"A doctor?" I laughed. "I'm too old!"

"No, you're not. And you would make a great doctor. But I think perhaps it might be even more helpful to write your stories."

"They hurt too much," I blurted honestly.

"Someday they won't hurt as much," he said, very gently. "Now is not the time. But there *will* come a time. There will be many, many more years for you to do many things, later."

Dr. Moore released my hand. "For after this," he said, "you still have a lot left to do."

· 31 ·

So What's a Geriatrician
and Why Should I Care?

$\mathcal{D}$r. Moore said one more thing. It was time for my mother to see a new physician. She would benefit from being followed by a geriatrician.

"See a new doctor? She likes you!" I replied. "And what's a geriatrician?"

Dr. Moore explained he was not suggesting the change because he didn't want to care for my mother anymore. Rather, it was because he felt a physician specializing in older people's health would provide the best medical treatment for her myriad conditions. I remembered suddenly that both Dr. Montgomery and Dr. Hobbs had been geriatricians. I recollected, too, how my father's medical treatment had dramatically changed for the better once they became involved in his care.

"A geriatrician is the expert for seniors," continued Dr. Moore. "They are internal medicine doctors like I am but have additional years of fellowship training specifically in old people's diseases. When it comes to age-related problems, these specialists are the most highly trained and up to date in procedures, understanding, knowledge, and treatment of conditions that affect the elderly. For these reasons, I would like to refer your mother to a fine geriatrician, Dr. Patricia Thompson."

"She will miss you," I said, hesitantly.

"Please understand I am happy to continue seeing your mother, if she prefers, but I think Dr. Thompson will have new insights into her complex health problems. In a perfect world, I truly believe every person over sixty-five should begin seeing a geriatrician. But they're getting harder to find."

"Why, if they are that important?"

"Because it requires years of rigorous study to become board certified in geriatric medicine, and it's far more profitable to be a dermatologist or a surgeon than it is a geriatrician or pediatrician. Added to that, geriatricians work

202

with old people. Most elderly are on Medicare or Medicaid; those reimbursements can barely cover a doctor's expenses."

After leaving his office, I thought about what Dr. Moore had said. That geriatricians were the doctors that you needed when you got old, but there weren't many of them. It all seemed a bit turned around to me. It struck me, too, that before too many years John and I and the rest of the *boomers* would be old and requiring care.

Something was wrong with the picture. I shuddered momentarily, recollecting a conversation I had with a nurse at the West Ridge. It had to do with Medicare reimbursement.

"It's lucky your mom has Elizabeth," she had warned a few days before my mother was discharged to go home. "Otherwise, she probably would never walk again."

The nurse explained something I had learned previously the hard way. Medicare paid for only a limited amount of physical and occupational therapy home care. After two, three, or possibly a few more visits, it stopped. It didn't seem to matter that, if continued, a patient might yet still walk and live independently.

Before leaving the West Ridge, I had asked the social worker why that was—why physical therapy was so limited, especially considering that everything I had read stressed the importance of keeping mobile, especially in the elderly. She merely shrugged her shoulders.

"Take it up with Medicare," she replied a bit cynically, "or better yet, take it up with the policy makers who dictate Medicare. I've never been able to figure out why the system will pay for a $25,000 heart stent procedure for a ninety-three-year-old patient with advanced Alzheimer's and maybe nine months to live but won't pay for routine home visits of a physical or exercise therapist to keep older people healthier and in their own homes. Go figure."

After my mother returned home, her progress accelerated, thanks in a large part to Elizabeth. She had devised an exercise regime that helped my mother regain some of her prior fitness level. My mother would never come back to where she had been before the latest episode, but she was improving, following Elizabeth's soft-spoken but unremitting demands that she daily practice her leg, arm, shoulder, hand, breathing, and walking exercises. Through perseverance, Elizabeth helped stem the slippery slope my mother faced after her hospitalization.

"I think," my mother quipped on an afternoon while waiting to be seen by Dr. Thompson, "I am beginning to despise the word 'episode.'"

It was her first doctor's visit since leaving the hospital and convalescent center. Understandably, she was nervous, and seeing a new doctor for the first time only added to her apprehension. And, to be honest, it augmented mine, too.

"How many episodes have I had now?" she asked, then, a little pathetically. "Did I just wear out Dr. Moore?"

"Of course not," I replied, not knowing whether that were entirely true.

So what did a geriatrician really know that Dr. Moore didn't? At first glance at Dr. Thompson's office, I found myself reflecting on one of Dr. Moore's comments. He was right; this geriatrician's office was definitely not the spacious, beautiful doctor's office of the dermatology clinic I had recently been in to have a mole removed. *That* place had live orchids of varying colors on the tables next to modern, stylish couches. Two large fish tanks were situated in the office, with dozens of exotic fishes colorfully swimming around to make one think of Hawaii. Artistic watercolors hung on walls painted soothing hues. Even the patients looked well heeled: there were fashionably dressed men and women reading copies of *The Economist* or the *Wall Street Journal* that they picked up from the waiting-room tables.

This geriatrician's office was decidedly the opposite. While admittedly clean and sporting new carpeting, touches like elegant orchids and watercolor paintings were sorely lacking. Most of the patients were elderly, and many slumped in wheelchairs. Few were outfitted in stylish designer fashions. Plus, the small lobby was crowded; certainly no room for even one small fish tank.

Judging just from appearances, I could see why physicians might want to become dermatologists, not geriatricians. The patients in Dr. Thompson's office looked sick, and, from what I could tell, all had suffered "episodes."

Upon meeting the physician, however, my prejudicial thoughts regarding the disparities of waiting rooms instantly vanished. From the first moment, Dr. Thompson's large smile, genuine warmth, and emanating compassion made me feel we were in the right place, with a doctor who really cared.

She was a fortyish, attractive woman with shoulder-length brown hair and steady gray eyes. Entering the examining room without a glance at me, she instead directed her attention to my mother and sat down in a chair close to her. Introducing herself, she first made certain my mother could hear, then spoke slowly and clearly. Even more, her tone was highly respectful.

Instantly, my mother responded by sitting up straighter.

"Tell me about yourself, Margaret," began Dr. Thompson, evincing what appeared to be keen interest in my mother's attempts to describe how she felt, who she was, what had just happened to her. As usual, my mother kept looking at me to intervene—as I usually did at these appointments—but Dr. Thompson expertly brought her back to her own self, encouraging my mother to express herself, not to have her words interpreted by me. The physician seemed not at all rushed, and before long my mother relaxed, reacting like she had known Dr. Thompson for a long time. The next thing she did took me by surprise. "Margaret, I'd like to see your feet."

While my mother obeyed by taking off her shoes, I was struck by the request, which sounded as if it were as routine as asking to listen to my mother's heart or checking her eyes. After examining her heels and toes, Dr. Thompson explained.

"Sore feet cause a lot of problems in older patients," she said. "Yours are obviously cared for. When people have long, untrimmed toenails or sore calluses, it often results in problems for them walking and can lead to a fall."

"I don't want to fall!" said my mother, quickly.

"I don't want you to fall, either," said Dr. Thompson.

Instantly I was thrown back to my father—how he insisted that his patients take care of their feet. How he put them in those early, funny running shoes. How he went to nursing homes every few weeks to volunteer his time trimming toenails and tending to painful feet. I remembered even then he had talked about the importance of keeping feet healthy to protect his patients from falling.

Dr. Thompson continued asking my mother lots of questions about her feelings. I could tell how quickly my mother was warming to her and observed how the skill of a physician trained in dealing with old people could help make an elderly patient divulge what they were really thinking and feeling. My mother had not bubbled so much to a doctor since Dr. Moore had called her "frisky."

Then, Dr. Thompson asked her a question that she had heard before. From my mother's expression, I knew she was reliving that awful déjà vu—that "here we go again" feeling—of when my father had been tested for Alzheimer's. The battery of questions and answers was the same, and we both remembered it too well.

"Margaret," said Dr. Thompson, "can you spell 'world'?"

My heart sank as I watched my mother's spirits deflate before my eyes. Frowning, she concentrated for a minute, looking at her lap and putting her hands together like a schoolgirl who's just been reprimanded.

She sighed. "W . . . O . . . L—I mean R . . . L . . . D."

Dr. Thompson did not congratulate her, nor even act like my mother had done anything she did not expect her to do. "Now, please spell it backward."

Oh God, I thought. Now I'm going to have to dive in and say that she can't do that, but really, she isn't too demented, even if she seems to be.

"D . . . L . . . R . . . um . . . O and W," said my mother.

"Thank you, Margaret; I have only a few more questions like this and then we can move on," said Dr. Thompson. She continued with the routine string of inquiries, but somehow, her kind tone didn't make them seem as depressing as usual. After she was through, she smiled at my mother.

"I think you are returning to more of your baseline," she said, and then, for the first time, directed her attention to me. "According to Dr. Moore's notes, your mother, when she was in the hospital, was not in the same condition as she had been only a few days before."

"The doctors there said she had advanced Alzheimer's," I remembered, wearily.

"She does not have advanced Alzheimer's."

"Does she have dementia?"

"That's what I'm trying to figure out." And then Dr. Thompson did a funny thing. She called in her nurse to take my mother to another room for blood work and a urinalysis. As she had already spent an hour with us, I stood up, figuring the appointment was through.

"Please wait for a moment," said the doctor to me. "There's some more I would like to go over with you."

And then she reserved the next half hour . . . just for me.

What I Wish I'd Known

The Tsunami Is Coming . . .
and Why *You* Should Be Worried

Elizabeth Eckstrom, MD, MPH, MACP

*E*very day, ten thousand people in the United States turn sixty-five. By 2030, there will be seventy million people over age sixty-five, or one out of five Americans. Today, sixty-five-year-olds can expect to live at least nineteen more years. The question becomes, what will life be like for those years? The answer: Research has proved that good geriatric care can make all the difference in your aging positively.

Studies show that when healthcare for older adults is overseen by a certified geriatrician as compared to traditional medical models, there are a number of important benefits. The most significant include (1) increased quality of life for older patients, (2) more years of independent living, (3) less time spent in the hospital or a nursing home, (4) lower "morbidity" (or presence of disease), and (5) lower death rates.

Geriatricians are medical doctors trained to deal exclusively with the problems and diseases of aging people. They are the counterpoint to pediatricians, who specialize in the care of children from birth to age eighteen. It takes many years of intense study to become a certified geriatrician. After four years of college, one must complete four years of medical school and then three years of a formal residency program in either internal medicine or family medicine. After that, one must enter into a one- to three-year fellowship program in geriatric medicine. The cost to become a geriatrician is high; student loans for medical school alone usually mount to nearly $200,000.

The specialty of geriatrics is complicated. Instead of patients coming in for one or two complaints, most geriatric patients arrive with multiple conditions. Many have between five to ten chronic ailments, such as heart disease, diabetes, or pulmonary problems. Simple cases are the exception. This means that a geriatrician must not only have knowledge and training about each individual problem but also understand and manage the *interactions* among them all.

The reason for much of the complexity is this: A body over sixty-five does not work the same way physiologically as that of a twenty-five- to forty-year-old. Various organ systems begin to suffer decline and do not operate as well or as efficiently. Also, the aging body responds to diseases differently and often reacts to medications much differently than if the same medications were used in a younger person. This can create a problem when a provider does not have additional expertise in geriatrics. Symptoms displayed by older people are often incorrectly diagnosed as *"just a product of growing old"* when, many times, the real trouble is what type or the sheer number of drugs they've been prescribed.

Geriatricians receive specialized training to distinguish among the intricate subtleties of what is normal in the aging process and what is not. They are vigilant about assessing problems that hasten aging's deleterious effects—some of which may not be technically called "medical conditions" and are often overlooked by practitioners who do not have specialized geriatric training. Symptoms that might not bother a middle-aged patient may ignite a life-threatening situation in an older person. For example, mild gastroenteritis can turn into severe dehydration in an older person. A low-grade fever can lead to confused thinking. Many commonly prescribed drugs can cause dizziness in older people. All three side effects—dehydration, unclear cognition, and unsteadiness—can have disastrous ramifications in older patients. Geriatricians understand that any one of those could predispose their patient to fall and break a hip. Each year, 350,000 people break their hips, with nearly half of sufferers ending up in a nursing home. Of those, 20 percent will never walk again.

The goal of geriatric medicine is to help patients remain *functionally independent* for as long as possible. Geriatricians want to keep their patients walking and able to manage *activities of daily living* such as dressing and feeding themselves. They strive to avoid nursing homes or hospitals. Geriatricians are fully aware of the high cost—physically, emotionally, and financially—of long-term care facilities. Over 50 percent of patients who move permanently into nursing homes use up their entire life savings, ending up on Medicaid to afford it.

To achieve these objectives, while realizing that not all conditions in older adults can be "cured," geriatricians look for holistic ways to improve their patients' lives. Different from traditional medicine, geriatricians often work in multidisciplinary teams to comprehensively care for their aging patients' unique physical, psychological, and social needs. Acting as the leader and care coordinator of the team, they work closely with other physicians, nurses, social workers, pharmacists, physical and occupational therapists, and others to help their patients have a better quality of life as they age. This creative model has been proved to greatly increase patient and family satisfaction as well as reduce rates of depression, decrease hospital and nursing home admissions, and preserve an older patient's physical function.

For all these reasons, Dr. Moore wanted Marcy's mom to be transferred to a geriatrician for specialized healthcare attention to optimize her remaining years of life.

Margaret was lucky. She found one. Most of us today, though, will not be so fortunate. At the same time as demand for geriatricians is on a trajectory to skyrocket, their availability is rapidly declining.

Since 1998, the number of board-certified geriatricians in the United States has dropped by over 25 percent to only 6,700. While people over eighty-five are the fastest-growing age group, numbering in the thousands, in 2012 less than one hundred doctors nationwide entered into geriatric fellowships. Current projections are that there will be only one geriatrician to treat every four thousand patients by 2030.

All across America, few new geriatricians are being trained. Why is this? One major reason is that geriatricians are among the lowest paid of any field of medicine, even though it requires years of specialty training. Most geriatricians are reimbursed solely by Medicare and Medicaid, and such low funding often cannot pay to keep an office running. Young doctors discover that even if they wanted to, going into geriatrics would not cover the costs of paying off their huge student loans. Subsequently, they need to find a different specialty. Many hospitals and clinics argue they cannot sustain keeping geriatricians on staff—citing that it is more profitable in terms of reimbursement to order a simple *wart removal* than for a patient to engage in an hour-long consultation with a geriatrician who needs to keep track of multiple issues to properly manage the patient's complicated health needs.

The future of geriatric medicine is in jeopardy, yet there is still another fact of major concern. Aside from geriatricians, most doctors today are not trained in how to appropriately manage elderly patients. *Ninety-seven percent of medical students in the United States do not take a single course in geriatric medicine.*

A crisis is brewing for those entering their senior years. Dr. David Reuben, a leading geriatrician at the UCLA Medical Center, is among the geriatricians who are worried about what this will mean to countless people on the cusp of aging. While the vast majority of Americans have no conception of what lies ahead, the fact that no trained geriatricians may be available to provide their healthcare will dramatically affect their lives.

"This is going to be the Hurricane Katrina of 2020," he says.

• 32 •

Pharmacopeia

$\mathcal{D}$r. Thompson led me to a small office with multiple plaques on the wall, a bookcase with papers and journals, and a large desk with a computer and more papers. The doctor sat down in her chair, and I pulled up a seat across from her. For a minute she didn't say anything but appeared to be deep in thought.

In time, I came to know this look of intense concentration. It was especially evident in the midst of any crisis. For Dr. Thompson never "reacted." She contemplated. And that act of mindfulness—pulling together her intelligence, medical knowledge, and insight—was a demonstration of fusing the true art and science of practicing medicine. As different nurses would tell me many times, when all other people would give up, Dr. Thompson would save lives.

The geriatrician asked me questions regarding my mother's health history and status in the past few years. She queried me about my father and his medical history as well. She reviewed again my mother's list of drugs she was currently taking.

Then she thought some more.

"Your mother does not have dementia, or, if she does, it is in early stages and a different type from what you saw with your father," she said.

I felt vast relief, but it was quickly tempered. "Then what was it that we saw when she was in the hospital? Another TIA?"

"No. What you observed was probably the worst, most frightening and heartbreaking thing anyone can see in a loved one. You experienced delirium."

She wrote down the words "delirium" and "dementia" on a piece of paper. "These are two entirely different things," she explained, "though they can be misdiagnosed or even mistaken for each other by a provider. Too often delirium is unrecognized."

"Why?"

"Because it can resemble dementia, anxiety, or depression. The key to delirium—like you saw—is that it typically manifests suddenly and severely. In your mother's case, I believe it was the result of an underlying and under-treated bladder infection and, in part, due to some of the medications she was on. I also suspect your mother may have another problem, common in the elderly—a REM sleep disorder. This can create bad dreams. Only now are we learning what a significant problem lack of restorative sleep can be for older persons. Like delirium, it often goes unrecognized and can cause great distress."

Dr. Thompson put down her pen and turned her steady, intelligent gaze on me. It wasn't sympathetic; it was factual, like she was talking to another professional.

"You were completely right to be so concerned," she said. "When delirium goes unchecked, the outcome carries a high cost. It can lead to serious medical problems and even death."

I thought of all the people in hospitals and nursing homes who had the same symptoms my mother had. What were *their* outcomes? Why didn't all providers and caregivers have the knowledge that there was a difference between delirium and dementia? Why did no one know about it—except, it seemed, geriatricians?

"There is an upside to all this," Dr. Thompson went on. "Whereas dementia is not reversible, delirium, when its underlying causes are appropriately treated, is."

Dr. Thompson pulled out my mother's pharmacy list and put it on the table between us. But she didn't talk about it just yet.

"Let me give you my thoughts as to what I believe is going on with your mother. She is very sensitive to delirium. When she suffers from it, she has huge swings. She can go from being great to being terrible . . . just as you witnessed. These swings are far greater than what they would be if they were from dementia. When your mother is in a downward swing from enduring a bad infection, she can become totally delirious. Additionally, she has hallucinatory delusions, like when she said she thought you were poisoning her."

For a few seconds, I relived that excruciating time once again. But now, with a name affixed to it *and* a reason, I saw it for what it truly was—a symptom.

"Additionally, I think the Charles Bonnet syndrome may also be an aggravation when your mother begins battling an infection. But there's something more."

Dr. Thompson took out her pen again. She displayed on the table a page listing all my mother's drugs. Next, before my eyes, she began crossing out one name after another!

"Here is a major problem," she recounted, still x-ing several more. "We call it *polypharmacy* or *pharmacopeia*."

From the expression on my face she knew I didn't have a clue what she was saying. She continued anyway. "Different specialists have prescribed your mother many drugs. Some are known to have adverse effects on the elderly. They can cause nausea, fatigue, or even hallucinations in a compromised older patient."

"Then why do doctors prescribe them?"

"Frankly, many providers don't understand the drug interactions that can go on in an old person. Part of the reason is that even the pharmaceutical companies don't really know. You see, most drug studies conducted on the efficacy or safety of these drugs, even commonly used ones, are done on middle-aged people, not senior citizens. Therefore, if you're not a geriatrician who studies this all day, most people don't realize the side effects of many routinely prescribed drugs on older, compromised patients." Dr. Thompson held up her pen. "Let's look at this list of what I've omitted."

Pointing at the page, she took each line item and explained her reasoning. "*Levaquin.* That antibiotic was prescribed for your mother initially for her urinary tract infection. That is a drug of choice for many people to fight infections. In the weakened elderly, though, especially those who are sensitive to delirium, it should never be used. It can cause hallucinations.

"Next, *Lipitor.* It can cause adverse reactions in an old patient," she continued. "In some susceptible patients, it creates muscle weakness and confusion. At your mother's age and after reviewing her cholesterol numbers, I believe we can safely discontinue it.

"Also, I am taking her off *Coreg* and *Lasix* for now. And," she tapped her pen to her notes, "here's another one. You mentioned that when she was in the hospital, they gave her this medication to help her sleep. You were correct in saying it seemed to jazz her up. It is contraindicated for the elderly and can do just the opposite of what you want it to."

Dr. Thompson turned her attention back to the printed chart. "Also, *Ambien*, which, from reading her chart, is a drug she uses on a regular basis for sleep, is not a good idea for her—at her age. I will prescribe another sleeping aid, *Trazodone*, that she should safely be able to use *on occasion* and in small doses. But I want to look into her sleeping problems more and try non-medicated treatments. And your mother should never be on *Phenergan* for nausea. I can prescribe a better drug that does not have the side effect of confusing her mental functioning."

As the physician continued explaining why she was discontinuing the majority of my mother's pharmaceutical regime, I was suddenly hit between the eyes with something I had never focused on before: the sheer number of pills my mother was taking every day. Imagine having to swallow all those! Just contemplating it was enough to make me gag.

Of course, I was familiar with all of the drugs—hadn't I made typed lists of them for all her caregivers, carefully noting which ones were to be given in the morning, which at noon, and then again at dinner, and at bedtime? Yet until this moment, I had never stood back to think how awful it must be to be prisoner of a marching army of drugs . . . like an unceasing offensive coming at you all day long, day after day, gaining strength in numbers, and going on—forever!

Witnessing Dr. Thompson at work, I deliberated about Dr. Moore's comments that all people needed geriatricians after they were sixty-five. Dr. Thompson obviously had a different "take" and understanding about health issues older people faced.

"What is often forgotten is that there is a *multiplier effect* to all these drugs older people are on," she continued explaining. "Their conglomerate interaction in an elderly individual can invoke many undesirable side effects. Old people's livers do not work as effectively as when they were younger to allow drugs to pass through and be excreted. What happens, then, is that these single remedies add up—like a large stockpile—one on top of the other. In effect, they are together creating one large super drug that an older person's body just can't deal with."

The illustration of all those daily pills glomming together in my mother's gut, and never being able to leave, was scary. How many old people's guts resembled my mother's?

"Drugs can do wonderful things, but too many can be deadly. Therefore, we need to be very careful about your mother's medications," Dr. Thompson concluded. "I think I have removed the most problematic ones, and I believe we should see a positive change in your mom's overall energy, mobility, and cognition."

By the clock, it had been one and a half hours. At last, Dr. Thompson stood up, and together we walked back into the examining room where my mother was sitting, thumbing through a magazine and looking at pictures. When Dr. Thompson came over to hold her hand to say good-bye and tell her she expected her to continue improving and feeling better every day, my mother seemed positively chipper.

"It's been a pleasure meeting you, and remember, Margaret, to keep working on those exercises now," said Dr. Thompson, exiting the room for her next patient.

My mother waited until Dr. Thompson had left. "Ugh," she breathed.

What I Wish I'd Known

Too Many Pills—The Fourth-Leading Cause of Death in Seniors

Elizabeth Eckstrom, MD, MPH, MACP

If medication problems were ranked as a disease, it would be the fourth-leading cause of death in older adults in the United States, after heart disease, cancer, and stroke. Complications related to too many drugs are a major problem and affect nearly one out of two senior citizens.

At the same time, clinicians often prescribe medications that have the potential to harm older patients. Without understanding the side effects, many providers treat certain conditions aggressively, despite a patient's age and functional status. What this means is that many people over sixty-five are at risk for "polypharmacy"—a dangerous situation.

What is polypharmacy, and why are people over seventy *seven times* more likely than a twenty- to twenty-nine-year-old to suffer adverse reactions to routinely prescribed drugs? How can you protect yourself or your loved ones from what researchers are calling a "significant cause of death in the elderly," but one that is entirely preventable?

Polypharmacy is defined as the concurrent use of several drugs—or consuming a number of drugs at the same time. This is a special problem for the elderly, for older patients take more medications than any other age group. Their panoply of drugs often includes medications for high blood pressure, constipation, high cholesterol, congestive heart failure, and diabetes, among others. On average, older persons take six prescription drugs plus three over-the-counter medications every day.

It is a problem that increases as you age. The older you get, the more drugs you are usually prescribed. But increasing the number of medications also amplifies the risk of serious drug interactions and unsafe side effects. Compounding the issue, frequently the side effects themselves are treated with even more drugs! Adverse consequences quickly multiply in relation to the increase in drugs consumed. When two drugs are taken, the chance of undesirable interactions is 5 percent. This percentage shoots to 100 percent when eight or more medicines are ingested per day.

Why are these reactions not "caught" before they become toxic? The answer is simple, yet disturbing. Many clinicians do not recognize the symptoms as being related to drug overuse because they *attribute them to an underlying medical problem or just being part of the aging process.* The most common adverse effects of polypharmacy include confusion, depression, fatigue, indigestion, dizziness, and urinary frequency. All of these can be erroneously dismissed by providers, family members, and patients themselves as *something that just happens when you grow old.*

This is often not the case. All older people and their families need to become vigilant to prevent the hazardous effects of polypharmacy from happening to them.

Why do drug side effects manifest themselves differently in older persons? It has to do with physiological changes and how drugs move in the body. The composition of an older body has less lean muscle mass, less water, and more fat. Because of this changing ratio of water to fat, some drugs have a longer "half-life," or a prolonged duration of action and higher drug concentration. This factor can produce a pronounced negative effect.

Also, the aging body has decreased liver mass (the liver is smaller) and reduced liver blood flow. Too, the kidneys do not work as efficiently. This means that the "clearinghouse" provided by the liver and kidneys to remove a drug from the bloodstream and body is diminished. Drugs that in a younger person would be metabolized and excreted instead build up and "stick around" in an old person. The risk of toxicity increases, as well as the probability of more serious side effects and "drug-drug" interactions.

Certain classes of drugs can cause adverse reactions in older adults and should never be prescribed yet, unfortunately, commonly are. Why? Most drug studies are conducted on younger people, and the side effects in older persons are not always known. Older persons routinely suffer toxic effects from doses that fall within the "normal range" for middle-aged patients. Beyond that, many drugs have not been studied *in com-bination,* so doctors don't know how serious the drug-drug interactions could be.

Indeed, as more drugs are studied in older people, more scientists are becoming aware of new and dangerous side effects of drugs in older adults.

Drug-drug interactions can lead to falls, illness, and death. However, these outcomes are usually preventable! One major study among nursing home residents found that 42 percent of all adverse drug reactions and a whopping 61 percent of life-threatening and fatal events associated with polypharmacy *were preventable.*

What does this mean to you or your parent? Foremost, be skeptical! Question your doctor about every drug you are taking and why is it necessary. And anytime a provider recommends starting a new medication, ask the following questions:

What is this drug for?
What side effects could it cause?
How will we know it's working?
When will the drug be stopped?
How will we monitor for side effects?
What other medications could this pill interact with, and how can
    I ensure that doesn't happen to me?

Also, make sure that any drug you are prescribed is not on the Beers list. This is a summary, created by geriatricians, of drugs that have been deemed extremely risky for older adults.

This list, with both generic and brand names noted, and the drugs' adverse effects, can be found in Appendix 1.

It is a good rule of thumb for older patients to review their entire medication list at every provider visit to see whether there is anything that is no longer needed or that could be given in a lower dose. Though you should never stop taking a drug without medical advice, be alert. Look for duplicate medications, such as generic and brand drugs. Make sure you are not taking two medications that are from the same drug "family." Remember, too, that even drugs that you have recently discontinued can still be in your body because "clearance" takes much longer in an older person, sometimes weeks.

Studies show that 17–25 percent of all hospital admissions in older adults are due to adverse drug reactions. Beyond that, older persons often experience adverse drug events when they *are* hospitalized because of even more drugs being prescribed there. Adding insult to injury, these patients are more likely to contract dangerous, antibiotic-associated *Clostridium difficile* infections (and others!) because of polypharmacy.

Minimizing medications is one of the best ways to avoid unnecessary emergency room visits, hospitalizations, and side effects. Older individuals are at a much greater risk of polypharmacy, especially if they have multiple healthcare providers or use more than one pharmacy. Communication between providers, attention to appropriate prescribing for older adults, and coordination of care is therefore paramount.

Polypharmacy is rampant in older adults and highly dangerous. Never assume any symptoms—such as mental confusion, insomnia, drowsiness, weakness, joint pain, exhaustion, or dizziness—in you or your loved one are merely a consequence of aging. *All older people need to maintain a healthy skepticism about any pills.* Keep drug-induced reactions in the front of your mind, and report any new symptoms you see at once to your provider. Check the Beers list. Be proactive and advocate for yourself or your parent.

Too many drugs can kill you. But if the effects of polypharmacy are caught early and appropriately intervened upon, you can help an older person return to better functioning. Even more, you may save your loved one's life.

• 33 •

The Search Begins

*J*ust as things were beginning to improve all around, there came another stroke of bad news . . . in fact, it was possibly the worst news I could imagine:

Alonzo was leaving.

After Inez's heart attack, he felt he needed to spend more time with her to look after her needs. On top of that, Mariana timidly gave more unfortunate notice: she was moving to California. Now began a scramble I had only heard about but never experienced: finding a caregiver for my mother.

No one wanted to really leave my mother; they all loved her. After ten years together, this was hard on all of us, for what Alonzo, Inez, and Mariana had done was more than just a job description. They had all become friends. Beyond that, they had become family.

I had heard horror stories about caregivers. It seemed at least once a week the paper would have an article about a caregiver who stole the old person blind, locked their client in a closet, or took the medications themselves. Some accounts were worse—caregivers who actually abused their clients or left them so long unattended and in filth that the patients developed bedsores and died.

These were the extremes, of course, but they were cause for alarm. Caregiving was such an important service—and an expensive one, too—that it was critical to find someone trustworthy, caring, knowledgeable, and with at least a modicum of medical background. Alonzo had always taken it upon himself to help train and oversee anyone else who took care of my mother. But he was too busy to do much of that now, being preoccupied with Inez's healthcare. The past two months while he helped my mother transition back home had been a struggle for him, though he never complained. I needed to find help—and right away.

219

The hospital and the West Ridge each gave me handouts of care agencies they referred patients to. Agencies, they said, did background checks for criminal records of their employees. Further references came from the providers themselves, at their discretion.

I scanned the names of the recommended caregiving agencies. Each one seemed a black hole, and each name gave me pause:

Tiny Worries.

Did that mean that their service gave you little anxieties?

Helping Angels.

Sounded too much like the client had died.

Warm Hands Warm Heart Caregiving Services.

My mother always said it was cold hands, warm heart. What did warm hands mean?

Helping Hands.

Too many hands.

Little Mercies.

I needed big mercies.

Home/Heart/Health/Hands.

Sounded like the 4-H pledge. And hands again.

Visiting Companions.

Sounded like a traveling pet service.

I decided, though, on Visiting Companions after talking to their representative, who said they had been in business for over twenty-five years and had excellent reviews from prior clients. The office manager informed me they had two seasoned caregivers with eighteen years of experience between them who could start right away. One had worked for ten years in hospitals and had CNA training. Would I like to interview them?

I set up two appointments at my mother's house after learning that other people my mother knew had experienced good luck with Visiting Companions. One daughter of a family friend said she had used the agency for both her parents until they died and never had a problem. They screened their workers well, and although they were slightly more expensive than some agencies, it was worth it for the peace of mind, she said.

Delores arrived first. Tall, in her early sixties, with graying blonde hair, the first thing I noticed about her was her hands. They were large, with big thumbs, and appeared strong and fully capable of lifting my mother from the bed or into the car. Her other attribute, while not a flaw, was more nettlesome. Every sentence uttered from her mouth began with the endearment "honey bunny."

"Honey bunny, it's a pleasure to meet you," she said at the door step, gripping my hand with her powerful fingers. Meeting my mother, she gushed,

"Honey bunny, aren't you too cute." But it was easy to see there was raw power behind the sweetness. Delores explained that most of her experience was at psychiatric hospitals with lockdown conditions. I responded that I didn't think she would have any of those kinds of problems with my mother.

Vicki came the following day for an interview. She was about the same age as Delores, but the similarity ended there. She had dyed, jet-black hair, black eyebrows penciled in the shape of two *U*'s, and false black eyelashes. Her lips were lined in red. She said she had been a beautician but discovered her true passion was taking care of old people. What sold my mother on her was her comment about nails.

"My favorite thing to do with the elders is to give manicures and pedicures," she smiled at my mother. "I have lots of colors you can choose from."

Visiting Companions maintained that both Delores and Vicki had fantastic references and, as a guarantee, if ever we were not pleased with them, the agency had a return policy that they would find a replacement to our liking.

"I'm not really sold on either of them," I told John honestly, "but what can I do? They have been screened and seem decent enough. My poor mom is going to go nuts, though, being called 'Honey' every other breath. Luckily, Delores wants to work evenings and nights when my mom goes to sleep."

"And the other one?"

"Vicki seems okay, though a little spacey."

"When is Alonzo leaving?"

"This weekend."

"Mariana?"

"Same."

"Then," said John, "I don't think you have much choice."

The following week marked the beginning in a new chapter of caregivers. I quickly realized I had been spoiled by Alonzo. For one thing, having two new employees and an agency to boot meant there was lots more paperwork. Costs were not just by the week or month but by the hour. Schedules were fixed; flexibility was not something I could count on.

Also, I knew it was important to be very clear about medications. I drew up a sheet detailing every prescription or vitamin or eye drop she was to have and at what time, and then I laminated it and put it on the refrigerator. One problem became clear right away, though—the dosage of Coumadin. My mother had to have her blood levels checked each week and her Coumadin doses adjusted accordingly. Some weeks the dose was four milligrams; others, two milligrams. Sometimes, if her blood was too thin, the Coumadin pill might be skipped for a day or even given every other day. What was critical was that my mother's blood was thinned to the "safe" margin. Discussion and clarity with the nurses was paramount; Alonzo had done the job flawlessly. But now, I knew, it would fall once more to me. It was too important to leave to chance.

Other tasks took time as well. Both Delores and Vicki needed to know the ropes of the house. Where the sheets were. How all the appliances worked. Where the keys were kept. Where my mother slept and which rooms she loved to be in. Which were the right buttons to push for the "stair glide" to the basement garage.

When my mother had been recovering at the West Ridge, I had a movable chair installed in her house on the advice of Elizabeth. She worried about the long flight of stairs that connected the living area of the house with the lower level, where the garage was located. In time it was becoming more difficult for my mother to negotiate them. Elizabeth suggested a company who could put in a stair glide so that my mother could ride up and down the stairs and not be concerned about falling.

My mother instantly loved the new device except for one feature: the seatbelt.

"Why do I need to be buckled in? I'm just riding down to the basement."

But Elizabeth and I agreed it would be too easy for her to lean forward or get up too soon and risk having a bad fall. My mother, though, always wanted to cheat and not wear it. She bristled at my insistence.

"I think your real calling was as a policeman," my mother said, exasperated after overhearing me expound to both Delores and Vicki that she must be belted in at all times when being conveyed on the stair glide.

A little glitch happened over starting dates. Delores was eager to begin work right away. Vicki said the timing would fit with her schedule too. But at the last minute, Vicki requested an additional week of vacation before coming to work full time. Her previous client had died only recently, and Visiting Companions called to say Vicki would prefer having one more week to grieve. Mariana graciously said she could put off moving during that time, and Alonzo agreed that the request showed that Vicki seemed a sensitive person, which was a good thing.

The actual transition between caregivers went fairly smoothly with the exception of Delores's militaristic manner in handling my mother. Delores liked set schedules . . . and rules. Not that my mother went out of her way to be naughty, but she was not fond of rigid timetables for her sleeping, waking, and eating times, and Alonzo had been good with that. Delores, though, with her background in psychiatric wards, was used to keeping clients on strict programs. This meant adherence to routines for bedtime. And in Delores's experience, this did not include the occasional nightcap.

"I'd like a glass of my Rhine wine tonight," my mother expressed to Delores one evening before going to bed.

"Honey bunny, dinner was two hours ago. It's sleepy time now, honey."

"Sometimes I don't want my wine at dinner," persisted my mother. "Some nights I prefer to listen to books on tape with a glass of white wine before I go to sleep."

"Honey bunny, you should have mentioned that earlier. Like I said, it's time for bed now, honey."

My mother phoned me at once. I could hear Delores breathing heavily in the background. Explaining the predicament, my mother handed Delores the phone, and we worked through that.

My mother got her wine.

But it wasn't Delores I was anxious about. She was tolerable, if not great. Delores liked to sleep ten hours, and my mother did too. Vicki, however, was a different story. The warning bells should have gone off right away, and, in a way, they did; I just didn't know enough to heed them.

The initial alarm came during Vicki's first full day at work. My mother had phoned to say that Vicki was very nice and had painted her nails. She didn't like the color, but Vicki said she would redo them tomorrow.

An hour later I received a second call. This time, not from my mother.

"Are you Margaret's daughter?" came a deep, husky voice, halting my heart. "This is Lieutenant Brady from the Cedar Crest Fire Station."

He continued on before I could erupt with questions. "I am standing here in the living room with your mother. A black-headed lady is with me and says she works for you. I just want to check things out."

"Is the woman's name Vicki?" I gasped.

"Your name Vicki?" I heard him ask and then a weak voice reply, "Yes."

"Why are you there, Lieutenant?" I broke in. "Is my mom okay? Has there been a *fire?*"

"No fire. Your mom's fine and wants to talk to you. But this lady showed up at our fire station a while ago and said she had locked herself out of the house. We drove her back, and your mom let us in. I want to make sure this story is for real, your mother being elderly and all."

I explained to Lieutenant Brady that this was Vicki's first day at work and thanked him for his assistance and caution.

Then I got in the car and drove right over to see what in the hell was going on.

• 34 •

Honey and Dummy

$\mathcal{V}$icki met me at the door in tears.

"Go ahead, fire me right now. I'm so stupid—stupid—stupid!" she wailed. "I didn't want your mom to stand up if I banged on the door. I was afraid she might get startled, get up, and fall."

"Banging on the door?" I queried, mystified.

She looked down, contritely. "Well, you see, I was outside."

It was October, dark and cold. "So just what were you doing outside?"

Vicki shuffled a foot, like she had just been caught doing something bad. "Um, well, smoking."

This *was* bad. I had specifically requested a caregiver who did not smoke. Vicki had lied and said she was a nonsmoker.

"But I'm trying to quit!" she blurted. "I am on Nicorette. When I get nervous, the gum doesn't do it. I knew you didn't want anybody smoking *in* the house. When I saw your mom was sleeping in her chair, I stepped outside. The French door is glass, and I could see your mom just fine. But after I finished, I realized the door locked from the inside."

My mother was listening and nodding; she seemed entirely sympathetic. It was then I noticed her brilliant orange nails.

More tears were rolling down Vicki's cheeks. "I was afraid to knock. What if your mom thought I was a burglar, trying to break in? I didn't know what to do!"

"So what did you do?"

"I didn't have your number or my phone with me, so I went out to the street," she confessed, breathlessly. "I started walking up and down the road. Finally a man in a car picked me up. He offered to drop me off at the fire station, about a mile away. Then Lieutenant Brady drove me here and called you."

Vicki wiped her face with a Kleenex she grabbed from a box next to my mother's chair. "I really wanted to do a good job today because your mom and I had fun. Right, Margaret? I did her nails, and she likes that. And now if you fire me, poor Margaret won't have anybody because Delores is quitting."

"Delores is *quitting*?"

"Yes," proffered Vicki. "She told me this morning when I came that it was too far for her to drive. The agency will be calling you tomorrow." Vicki glanced at my mother with poignant eyes. "I can't tell you how sorry I am. I promise, if you keep me on, this will never happen again!"

Without Delores or Vicki I was stuck between the proverbial rock and hard place. The only positive thing was that Vicki appeared to be honest. At least she owned up. After a few moments of contemplation, I replied, "I'm not going to fire you."

"Really?" Vicki raised her orange, fake nails—the same hue as my mother's—to her mouth in a gesture of disbelief. "You are so, so kind!" she cried. "For *you*, I am going to give up smoking forever!"

"George never liked smoking," added my mother. "He said it was bad for your health."

I held back my smile while Vicki continued drying her eyes.

Later that night, when John heard the story, he disagreed with my decision to keep Vicki on.

"In most cases, I'm forgiving," he said, thoughtfully. "But when it comes to your mother's care and safety, I wouldn't be."

"Oh, Vicki's harmless," I retorted. "She's just made one blunder, and she's sorry. And she promised to never smoke again."

John was not convinced. "It's not the smoking I'm worried about. It's her judgment. It's up to you, of course. But if it were me, I'd fire her. I would err on the side of 'one strike, you're out.'"

"But I think she has a good heart," I came back, to Vicki's defense.

"We'll see," he said, then dropped it.

It was only later . . . much later . . . that I deeply regretted my choice. Not only did I end up giving her one strike, but, in the end, four. The last one nearly killed my mother.

But in all my years of caregiving, I never saw it coming.

Visiting Companions didn't contact me the following day to tell me about Delores's decision to quit. Not wishing to wait, I called the office manager myself to advise them to begin a new search. But the manager sounded surprised, saying Delores had never broached the topic with her. It was a little bit odd, but I chose to overlook it, reasoning that Delores probably mentioned something to Vicki about resigning and then changed her mind.

I also was prepared to overlook another "Vicki event" that happened the next month. Alonzo, though, when he heard of it, went through the roof.

"No—no—no!" he shouted. "A caregiver should never bring a strange man into your mother's home!"

I tried to explain that it wasn't a strange man. It was Vicki's fiancé.

"No matter," chastised Alonzo. "He doesn't work for you. He should not be in her home. I don't like it one bit."

John didn't either. But again, I rationalized for Vicki. I had discovered the man sitting in my mother's den one day when I popped over for an unexpected visit. Vicki, embarrassed, testified that her fiancé was only there to help move some books my mother had asked to be brought from the den to the living room. "Lennie is strong," said Vicki. "I didn't think anyone would mind."

I immediately told her that I did not want anyone else there unless I gave prior permission. Once more, she was repentant and promised it would never happen again.

"You believe her?" reproached Alonzo. "Your mother can't see. How does she know if anyone is there and who they are? I don't trust—Lennie."

Actually, I didn't really either, especially after being warned by both John and Alonzo, but it was my mother who blamed herself over the whole ordeal.

"I think I remember telling Vicki that Lennie could come over," she said. "I wanted to meet him. You know, Vicki's love life is really like a movie. She's had so many disappointments. She told me that Lennie is the dream man she has been waiting for all her life."

She was obviously more enamored with Vicki's running soap-opera dialogue than concerned with her lapses in good sense.

"—And now they are talking about picking out rings," said my mother. "She's asked for my advice."

Caregiving skills aside, Vicki kept my mother entertained. I decided to let the matter drop as long as Lennie didn't show up again.

But the next happening was far more serious. After Vicki had been on the job for less than three months, she phoned, with a frantic tone in her voice. "I think I may have just done something stupid."

"What now?" I started to say but caught myself.

"I thought I was doing you a favor. On Monday afternoon, the Coumadin nurse called to say your mother's dose had changed. I know it's a lot for you to have to continually drive over and put the new dose into the pill cases. So I decided to do it for you."

"What did the nurse say it was?" I asked, growing nervous.

"She said your mom was to have four every day for the rest of the week."

"Four milligrams," I interjected quickly. "That's *one* tablet. *Each tablet* is four milligrams."

"Ooooooo. I guess I shouldn't have . . . then," Vicki sighed.

"Shouldn't have what?"

"I thought that meant four *pills*," choked Vicki.

"So what have you been doing?" I stammered.

"I've given her four pills of Coumadin for the last three days. They're big and kinda hard to swallow—"

"What? You've been giving my mom *sixteen milligrams of Coumadin for the past three days*?"

"Is that what it adds up to? I'm really sorry."

Oh my God, I thought. My mother could have a major bleed. "Don't move her," I said quickly. "I'm calling the doctor."

"But we were just on our way out to the store—"

"No! This is quite serious, Vicki," I cried. "Stay put."

Slamming the phone down, I cursed myself and Vicki for the mistake. Then I called both the doctor and the Coumadin clinic. They got back to me rapidly, saying my mother needed vitamin K immediately to counteract the dangerous effect of repeated quadruple doses of the blood thinner. Additionally, a visiting nurse was sent out to come to the house and check my mother's blood levels.

I called John and told him the news and that I wouldn't be able to make the high school senior meeting this afternoon. I had to find vitamin K.

Locating a source for vitamin K was harder than I expected. No one, aside from our veterinarian, who carried it for pets that digested d-CON, seemed to have it in stock. Several hours passed before I found a place and an hour more before I got it to my mother, who had no idea she had just been inadvertently poisoned by her caregiver.

The visiting nurse confirmed my mother's blood levels were out of a safe zone and the vitamin K was imperative. They would keep an eye on her. After the nurse had left, Vicki wrung her hands as she apologized to me in the kitchen.

"I'm just thankful you called me, Vicki," I said, seething inside. "You know you aren't to interfere with my mother's medications. I do the dosing."

"Oh, I know, I know! I won't mess with your mom's meds ever again!" she promised. "I just wanted to help. You've been looking real tired lately, and you've got that rash on your neck. You probably can't see it, because it's on the back."

"There's no rash," said John, later, when he got home and I made him look. "Vicki's seeing spots and probably should have her eyes checked. How's your mom?"

"Fine, but I feel terrible! These things never happened with Alonzo! Last week Vicki cut my mother's catheter in two when she cleaned it. The visiting nurse had to come back then as well and put in a new one. Will it ever end? I'm just an awful caregiver!"

"Not you; Vicki. You're a good caregiver. And that's not the problem."

"Then what is the problem?"

John tenderly wrapped his arm around me. How was it that he could always see what was wrong, settle my soul, and somehow then put everything right?

"Your problem, Mar," he said, handing me a napkin for the tears he knew were coming, "is who you have working for you. Remember Goofus and Gallant? You've hired *Honey and Dummy*."

• 35 •

Mountains and Valleys

$\mathscr{I}$ put the phone back in the receiver and sat down. Then I placed my head in my hands. No one was home. No one could hear me.

Taking a deep breath, from the bottom of my stomach, I screamed.

I was going to have to miss yet another school function—one I had been long looking forward to. Jennifer was a senior in high school, and today was her last parent-teacher conference. There was also an art show, and her painting of a mountain lake in the Wallowas had been selected to be prominently displayed near the school's entrance.

Once again, I would disappoint her and not be there—just like I had let down Emily when she had her senior choir concert and Nana was in the hospital. I had missed numerous soccer games and science fairs. Why? Because it seemed I was always *dealing with some emergency* or, like today, because the *caregiver had to leave* and someone had to take my mother to her damned dermatology appointment.

That made me feel guilty, too. Shouldn't I want my mother to find relief?

Delores had called with the news that my mother continued to be afflicted with "itching"—a malady she'd had for the past few weeks. My mother was scratching herself raw in places and, as Delores explained, "She won't keep her fingernails off her arms and legs, even when I threaten to handcuff her!"

I knew my mother was truly miserable, and in the past few weeks we had been to several doctors, but to no avail. Even Dr. Thompson's prescribed ointment was unsuccessful in curtailing the problem. Today's appointment with a dermatologist was her final hope. Only yesterday she had called me in a fit of desperation.

"My rash is getting worse. If I don't get some sort of cure, I don't think I want to keep on living."

Delores reconfirmed my mother's agitation with a negative prognosis of her own.

"I think you're mom's going crazy," she said, knowingly. "She's going to scar herself silly." Delores added she'd had some patients, when she worked at the mental hospital, who had scratched themselves to bleeding due to psychological disorders.

Just before getting off the phone, she added that she wouldn't be able to take my mother to her appointment today. She felt ill.

"What about Vicki?" I asked.

"I already called her. She's busy doing something with Lennie. Your mom, though, she needs to have her hands bound. Sometimes patients act like they're going to kill themselves with scratching."

That was a bad idea. Who would have thought that a simple ailment such as itching could have such devastating consequences? That left no one to go with her except me.

After trying to settle my disappointment, I called John. He said not to worry. He was planning on attending the art show and conference and would hold down the fort.

But it wasn't that I wanted the fort secured, I felt like shouting back. I wanted to be there!

All those caregiver manuals said there would be moments like this, I thought bitterly. Then they said all you needed to do was take care of yourself.

Baloney. There wasn't time to take care of yourself! And if you did, then you felt guilty for that too.

The bottom line was something that no book was telling you. So much of the time, at least for me, I felt I was letting *everyone* down.

The self-help books on dealing with aging parents talked about ways to "recharge" yourself. Well, I knew them all by heart and did most of them routinely. I ran or exercised most days, even if for a half hour. I kept a journal. (I *had* to do that; it stabilized me.) I went to church regularly. I attempted to meet, whenever possible, with good friends for support. I toiled (with mediocrity) at my job. I took walks outside. I felt grateful for my family.

The methods did help to equalize my emotions, but they failed in one major aspect: they couldn't reduce the *load*. The work I was doing was cumulative. And, one point the books never disclosed—all those things you did for yourself? They required effort and some discipline, too.

Right now, considering I was going to miss out once again on something that meant a lot to me, I was sick of acting disciplined. I wanted to tell the world, "No more am I going to paste on that sappy, happy face! From now on, you'll see the real me!"

But then those tiny portholes to my soul began letting in the dribbles of guilt, like a flashlight shining through a dark window. Just what kind of daughter was I? If people could see through the windows into my mind and heart right now, they'd be shocked. Peeking in, they would expect to see a loving heart saying: "Dear mother, we are going to the dermatologist! She will make you better! And then you'll be happy and want to live again!"

But that wasn't the scene roiling inside. Rather, a different voice was griping:

"Itching? *Itching*? What is the big deal about *itching*?"

If they peered a little longer, they'd see even more.

"Why should itching and scratching take up so much of your time and my time? My friends are doing lots of exciting things, and you and I are sitting here moaning about itching. How boring is that? Marie—you know her—is going with her parents and her two children to Antarctica! Susan is planning a trip this summer with her parents and kids to Africa, where they're going on a safari. And over winter break, Alex is taking her daughter to Disneyland."

The light was now blazing through the porthole, exposing the bald truth. "I want to do more for my children than itching and scratching. But I can't. Vicki I must watch like a hawk, and Delores wants to incarcerate you in an institution. My life is a failure. I am a failure. A failure as a mother. A failure as a daughter. A failure as a writer. And maybe even as a wife."

After another belly-emptying scream, I picked up my car keys, drove to my mother's, and took her to the dermatologist. Thankfully, the doctor said her condition was a singular form of eczema and was treatable. She prescribed my mother a new ointment that almost immediately provided relief.

Vicki came at seven, and I was able to go home. We had dinner, talked about the conferences and art exhibit, and Jennifer left to do her homework in her room. Then John cornered me to ask what in the world was wrong with me today.

"You can tell?" I asked. Then, all the pent up frustration came out once again on the one I loved the most.

John listened thoughtfully. "You need a break, Mar."

"Oh, yeah. How's that going to happen?" I said, cynically. "There are no days off for this job. And it's a job, job, job! What's more, I'm a pathetic failure at my job!"

John didn't disagree with my assessment. He waited until I started running out of steam before speaking.

"I think," he said at last, "the hard part of what you're doing isn't all the time you are putting in. And it's not even the work itself."

"What do you mean?"

"I think it's because, on some level, you understand that everything you are doing for your mother will ultimately fail."

I was confused. "Well, that's hopeful."

"No, Mar, this is what I mean. In the end, your mother is going to pass away. No matter what you do, or we do, nothing can stop that trajectory. She is nearly ninety, and none of us can live forever. You are seeing sad reflections of that fact day after day. And all of your continual efforts to change that course *can't*."

He was touching a chord I didn't want to feel. It was brutal yet burned with the hot flame of honesty.

"Your expectations to keep her alive forever are not realistic," he said. "*You* aren't the failure, Mar. You are, though, feeling the pain of failure."

I opened my mouth to reply but couldn't. John was right.

But it also helped that in the upcoming weeks, my mother's rash healed and her itching went away. Having her well for a time effectively removed a lot of the present anxiety. Taking advantage of the situation, and as it occurred over a school break, we arranged to take a family trip to the mountains for the weekend. Having my family around me and hiking in the alpine country did wonders to dispel the gloom I'd been feeling. When I returned and saw my mother's joyous smile beaming at me, I found I again could return it heartfully, genuinely, and with much love.

The dramatic change in my outlook was so pronounced that I found myself asking: What had made the change? And what could I do to protect myself from falling into that pit of despondency again?

On a sunny winter afternoon when I had a free moment, I decided to tackle the question. Grabbing up my journal, I threw on my down coat and headed outside to thrash out the matter. I sat down in the field, to the surprise of the sheep, who were munching on the short, late-season grass. A flock of sandhill cranes was crooning sonorous calls in an adjacent pasture. A mature red-tailed hawk dipped down in its flight overhead toward the river.

Taking out my pen, I began to write.

If I were ever to compose a caregiver's manual, I began, I would tell the truth. The fact of the matter is: it is vitally important to take time to *detach from caregiving!*

I thought back to the mountains. It didn't matter whether you had other caregivers or not. Or even whether your loved one was in a nursing home. Planning even short weekends away was critical to keep from burning out. You needed to carve time to physically remove yourself from the whole situation, and—here was the critical part—*leave the guilt at home*. You needn't worry; it would still be there when you returned. But it would be markedly reduced, leaving you more effective and renewed.

It was so important that I wrote it down twice: *It's not only okay, but crucial to take time away!* You need time to replenish yourself . . . to revive your heart! By detaching for a time, you will be energized to give your loved one a higher quality of care when you return.

It sounded contradictory, but it wasn't. By planning and taking routine short-term breaks, my mother would be receiving more, not less, of me.

But there was a second part, too. And perhaps it was the most important thing of all. Because, I realized suddenly, there was a trap that could ensnare you, not just once, but over and over. It had to do with your perspective. It was easy to get it wrong. And it was vital to get it right. I picked up my pen again: *Taking care of my parents is not a job. It is a journey.*

That slight shift in thinking made all the difference.

I thought back to the itching and scratching, to when my mother called me Shelby, to Dr. Hip, to Alonzo and Vicki, and to Eleanor and even Red-Eyed Ruthanne. It *was* a journey, with all its ups and downs, and we were on it together as a family. Of course, there was guilt—especially when it concerned my children and the fear that I was letting them down or denying them things (like trips to Disneyland) that other children may or may not have had. That, however, was not really the issue. In fact, it only masked it. What was important was the realization, the awareness, that there were hidden opportunities in our own expedition.

Through the crises that sometimes arose, we were given the chance to see life as it was in *real* time, not by the green-screen backdrops of fantasy. Along the way, my mother and father were showing all of us what it meant to endure problems and suffering with grace. Over the years, Emily and Jennifer were developing qualities of character, courage, and compassion that, in the long run, would serve them well. For all of us, it was a trip of endurance through mountains and valleys . . . a test of grit and faithfulness. This was our family's journey—with each other and for each other.

I placed my journal on the ground and stood up. Catching sight of the hawk again, I realized something starkly.

This was *not* the definition of a failed life.

The Care and Maintenance of Caregivers

Elizabeth Eckstrom, MD, MPH, MACP

Caregiving is hard. I have seen hundreds of family caregivers suffer as Marcy did, and the sad thing is that it is so difficult to find support and relief. Many caregivers never even allow themselves to think the things Marcy said. And no one enters a caregiving relationship with a family member knowing what might lie ahead—or with enough expertise to manage every situation that arises. Most people become a caregiver because they love their family member, because there really is no other option, and despite having a plate that is already plenty full. Maintaining health, happiness, and important relationships while caring for a frail loved one requires diligence, self-reflection, and humor—and occasionally taking the time to appreciate a soaring raptor. Here are some tips that may help ensure success in your caregiving journey.

1. Find your "team." Who are the people who will keep you sane—who will honestly tell you when you are at your wits' end, who will be willing to talk at midnight when you are exhausted from yet another crisis or when you are frightened to death because Mom is back in the hospital? Your sister? A close friend? A clergy? A counselor? Be willing to tell these people what is happening in your life and that you need them to be part of your team. *Not* sharing will lead to trouble down the line because it will be harder and harder to confess when you need a break, when you need a day "off," or when you truly need to escape for a while.

2. Develop a self-care plan. Write down your goals for self-care activities, such as exercise, spending time with friends, gardening, playing piano, and other things that rejuvenate you, and then keep a calendar to ensure you are doing them. When life gets hectic and you find you haven't done any self-care for a few days, stop and think about what needs to change to get back to your plan.

3. Remember that your first job is *not* to be a caregiver but to be a family member! If you are spending all your time taking your mom to doctor's appointments, getting her needed supplies and medicines, and helping her bathe and dress, you won't have any energy left for a loving relationship with her. Lots of family members feel guilty hiring caregivers to fulfill these menial tasks—they think it is their duty to care for their loved one's every need. But it is much more important to be fully able to *enjoy* your time spent together. Your mom doesn't want to remember you as always being frazzled, grumpy, and tired—she wants to remember the laughter, stories, good books, and relaxed lunches you are able to share. Your family member's physical needs can be met by another caregiver—no one else can provide the emotional support and love that you can. This is a treasure to be protected and fostered.

4. Take time to reflect—is this really the best me? If not, why not? Don't be ashamed if you think you aren't doing a good job—after all, were you trained for this job? Is this truly your area of expertise? Of course not. Take notes of what you've learned along the way so that you can become more expert—and then pride yourself on how well you handle tough situations. There will be days when you just wish your loved one would die so that it could all be over—this feeling is another clue that you need some respite; not a "bad" emotion that you have to push to the darkest recesses of your mind. Recognize that part of your feeling is grief over the loss of your younger, healthier parent and that it is best to grieve consciously, but also find the positives that are still left. When Marcy came back from some much-needed time away, she was able to enjoy her mom's beautiful smile again—and this made it all worthwhile.

5. Watch for red flags that your health is suffering. Ask a family member or friend to be observant too, and be sure to see your doctor regularly. If you develop headaches, fatigue, pain, abdominal problems, or other vague symptoms, these might be your body telling you that you are doing too much. Many caregivers become depressed, so watch for signs of depression such as lack of energy, trouble with sleeping or eating, or finding that you don't enjoy spending time with friends and family or doing things you usually love.

6. Be realistic about the expectations being placed on you. Often no one seems to realize that you spend hours every day caring for your loved one—and then still have to juggle your job, kids, house, and everything else. No one else is going to come to your rescue—so you have to be able to let others know when you are overwhelmed. And too many people think, "Oh, it is hard now, but it will get better, and I will be okay." Rarely do caregiving needs go down—rather, they keep going *up*. Start planning early for how you will get help beyond what you can provide. And talk with your parent's provider about what community services might be available—if your parent qualifies for Medicaid, he or she may be able to get some in-home or short-term respite care covered by Medicaid. If not, look to other community resources, such as the state-sponsored Area Agency on Aging, the long-term care ombudsman (if your parent is in a facility and things are not going well), the Alzheimer's Association, and other community organizations that might be able to help. Your local senior center will often be able to provide some assistance in finding the resources you need too.

No one has to survive caregiving alone, and no one *can* survive caregiving alone. If you are proactive about establishing your network of support, a self-care plan to keep healthy, and a reflection process to recognize caregiver burnout early, you and your loved one will enjoy a fuller, more gratifying relationship.

And in the end, as difficult as it is to accept this truth, your parent will die, which is *not* a failure on your part. By facing this inevitability, your caregiving objective becomes more clear: its highest goal is to try to make this culminating stage of your relationship as rich, as loving, and as rewarding as possible.

· 36 ·

Who's Taking the Trazodone?

My mother's sleeping prescription, Trazodone, needed yet another refill. Once more I took the empty bottle to the pharmacy. Even Phil, the pharmacist, mentioned that my mother must be having real difficulty sleeping at night. Dr. Thompson was concerned, too, but Vicki said that my mother was a nighthawk without the drug.

"I think she's getting her days and nights mixed up," offered Vicki. "Delores thinks so too. We agree your mom needs Trazodone or she won't sleep a wink."

Delores and Vicki had switched schedules on certain days, and half the time Vicki stayed with my mother at night. When I sometimes arrived to visit early in the day, I often found both Vicki and my mother fast asleep.

At times I wondered whether some of the disappearance of the pills was due to Vicki's occasionally popping one, but when I asked her, she was incensed. "You don't trust me; you're accusing me; and I'm only doing my very best! Why would I ever take a Trazodone?"

But regardless of how many were being consumed, I didn't like how drugged up my mother often seemed in the mornings. She defended the use of the sleeping pill, however, saying it was impossible for her to doze otherwise.

"I worry at night," my mother confided. "When I try to fall asleep, I can't help thinking about lots of things. And then I wake up in the middle of the night, even with Trazodone, and can't fall back to sleep."

John still blamed part of my mother's problems on Vicki. He said it was easier for her just to knock out my mom with drugs, and then she didn't have to work so hard. Plus, Vicki wasn't any fun. She never did anything with my mother. In his words, Vicki was a total bore.

"Delores isn't much better," I responded. "Her hands look like a man's, and she's tough, even if she does call my mom Honey Bunny."

"I disagree. And, unlike someone else, she's not cold hearted and mean," said John.

"Vicki isn't mean."

"I've always told you I think she has a mean eye. I don't trust her."

"Then what can I do?" I said, getting riled. "I can't go over there every day and cheer up my mom. She's getting more and more down. The girls aren't as available as they once were. They're busy now with their own lives—with Emily in college and applying to medical school and Jennifer about to graduate from high school. We're all overtaxed. On top of that, all of my mom's friends are dying! I'd be depressed too!"

Just the week before I had received word that my mother's very best friend—whom she had known since college—had died unexpectedly of pneumonia. I still hadn't been able to break the news to my mother. It was too close to the anniversary of my father's death, four years ago, and my mother already seemed down in the dumps. Milestones, I had discovered, could be times for wounds to resurface. On the anniversary of this one, for whatever reason, she was especially forlorn.

April 6 was cool and cloudy when we visited the cemetery. My mother had purchased a beautiful bouquet of Easter lilies that she carefully laid on the grass next to my father's headstone. "How can it already be four years?" she reflected. Then, after spending some quiet minutes without speaking, she turned with reluctance to head back to the car.

Just before reaching it, however, she whisked her walker around.

"What are you doing?" I asked, surprised.

"I need to go back."

A little mystified, I followed behind her as she purposefully maneuvered her walker back to the headstone. Stepping aside from the device, she leaned over my father's grave to reach her hand into the lilies, from whence she pulled a perfect flower.

"I nearly forgot; he wanted me to take this," she said, showing me the pure ivory Easter lily she held in her hand. Her eyes were moist. "He is giving it to me."

The early spring chill made it difficult to stay long outside, and once back in the car, I turned on the heat, preparing to take her home.

"I've been thinking," she said, clutching the lily close to her chest. "I don't like the arrangement. In fact, it has been keeping me up nights worrying about it."

"What? The flower arrangement?"

"I don't want to be on top," she stated.

"On top of what?"

"On top of Daddy. I know I shouldn't care and it sounds silly, but we only have one burial plot right now. When I go, the cemetery is planning to put my body on top of his. I don't want to be on top of him."

My mother was not joking; instead, her expression was deadly earnest.

"He won't . . . really . . . know," I suggested.

"But *I* will. I never slept that way in over sixty years of marriage. If they bury me there, I know I'll *never sleep well again after I'm dead!*"

The whole matter was upsetting her so much that I took her directly to the cemetery office. They seemed understanding. Perhaps they had experienced this kind of thing before. They wrote up an order for another plot right next to his . . . for a nice fee.

I began growing worried over my mother's increasing depression. Before my father had died, that had never been her nature. Friends with parents in similar situations gave me advice for other options, saying that perhaps what my mother needed was a change of scenery. Had I considered assisted living? A foster care facility? Adult day care? I would always reply that she loved her own home. She had lived there for nearly fifty years. All her memories were there. Her touchstones. She was aging in place, where she wanted to be.

Still others suggested what she needed was Paxil or Zoloft. One acquaintance said that she instructed her mother's caregivers to ply the antidepressants. And, of course, keep up those sleeping pills.

But a side of me was concerned about giving more and more drugs, especially after Dr. Thompson advised against it. After I discussed the matter with her, Dr. Thompson said she was not keen on antidepressants and the Trazodone was apparently not effective. The doctor said she wanted to stop the merry-go-round of its refills.

I told Vicki that we were discontinuing the Trazodone without further notice. While we were awaiting word of Dr. Thompson's new plan, I would come over and pick up the rest of the bottle of pills and dispose of them. But when I arrived two days later, Vicki said she'd searched and searched for the bottle but couldn't find it.

"I thought the Trazodone was right in your mother's bathroom," Vicki said, wide eyed. "I wonder if Delores moved it? Do you think she *took* it?"

"It was full," I reminded her. "I just refilled it."

"I'll ask Delores and keep looking," Vicki replied.

But Delores didn't know anything, and my mother said she had no clue; she only took what they gave her.

"I know what happened to the Trazodone. You do, too," John said. I stared at him. Was he intimating someone stole it? "The answer," he said, "lies with someone, besides your mother, who is groggy every morning."

What I Wish I'd Known

How to Get a Good Night's Rest—Naturally

Elizabeth Eckstrom, MD, MPH, MACP

$\mathcal{W}$e all have had nights when we've tossed and turned and felt fuzzy, lethargic, and cranky the next day. And the older we get, the more elusive a good night's rest seems to be. So it is not surprising that Marcy's mom, and even Vicki the caregiver, might be hopeful that a sleeping pill such as Trazodone might help. In this chapter, we will talk about what changes with sleep as we get older, how we can continue getting restful sleep as we age, and lastly, why sleeping pills can be some of the most dangerous poisons out there—and should be avoided.

WHAT IS DIFFERENT ABOUT SLEEP IN OLDER ADULTS?

When we are young, we typically sleep deeply and well for many hours. Scientists think this is because we need sleep to help our developing brains and bodies. In addition, we aren't yet troubled with the weight of the world and so don't need to lie awake stewing—like Marcy's mom admitted to doing. We spend many hours per night in the deepest stage of sleep (stage 3) and have few or no awakenings. However, as we get older, we spend more of the night in lighter stages of sleep (stages 1 and 2) and experience more nighttime awakenings. This is normal, and it is no cause for concern. The number of hours we sleep also changes dramatically as we age. It is normal to sleep as many as eleven hours per night as a kid. It is also normal to sleep as few as six hours per night as an older person. Yet often we *expect* that our older-age sleep patterns should be exactly as they were when we were younger. We wake up a couple of times in the night and immediately begin to worry that we won't get back to sleep. What happens then? We are wider awake and anxious and starting to get cranky already. We have predisposed ourselves to having no chance of getting back to sleep.

It is important to realize that sleep patterns undergo change as we age. When we get older, our patterns shift a little earlier in the night. This is called our "clock"—and it is a surprisingly tough bedfellow. When we are teens, we prefer to go to bed at 2:00 a.m. and sleep till 11:00 a.m. (I have always wondered why high school starts before 10:00 a.m.). During our working years, we usually may sleep from 11:00 p.m. to 6:00 a.m.—which is already an earlier pattern than we had as a teenager. As we enter our older years, we find we might want to go to bed at 9:00 p.m.—a change, but completely normal. Remember, though, we also might need to sleep only six or seven hours per night, so if we go to bed at 9:00 p.m., we might be up and ready to go at 3:00 a.m.! Most older adults don't think it is "right" to get up at 3:00 a.m., so they lie in bed another four hours. The next morning they complain they had a terrible night.

One of our jobs as we get older is to *adjust our expectations* for our sleep patterns. We should not expect to sleep as many hours as we used to and, beyond that, should not always count on sleeping through the night. This is totally normal.

WHAT SHOULD I WORRY ABOUT IF MY PARENT OR I START HAVING TROUBLE SLEEPING MOST OF THE TIME?

While our sleep routines indeed may change quite a bit as we get older, it is important to recognize when there is something truly wrong with our sleep. Many medical problems can impair sleep—such as obstructive sleep apnea, restless limb syndrome, depression, and heart disease, among others. If new memory troubles, high blood pressure, headaches, or excessive daytime sleepiness emerge at the same time that sleep difficulties seem to be worsening, a visit to the doctor is in order. In these cases, a medical problem may be causing poor sleep. Some medications also cause trouble. Drugs for high blood pressure, depression, dementia, cold symptoms, and others can create sleep problems. If difficulty sleeping is becoming more pronounced, it is well worth reviewing all medication usage with your doctor to see whether any of them could be the culprit.

HOW DO I ENSURE THAT I GET
THE BEST NIGHT'S SLEEP POSSIBLE?

Achieving a good and restorative night's rest involves three key remedies. None of these involves prescription drugs, and all are proved to be highly effective:

1. *Get good and tired!*

The one surefire way to be sure to get a good night's sleep is to be *good and tired*. When we were kids and before the advent of video games, we spent our entire day outside—running and playing and reluctantly coming in when Mom called bedtime. Guess what? We slept great. But by the time we are seventy, eighty, or ninety, we are not spending our entire days running around and playing anymore. Conversely, we spend most of our time sitting and watching TV, reading, napping, or sending emails to our grandchildren. What this means is that we have reduced our opportunity to find ourselves *good and tired* in the evening.

Our bodies were made for movement—movement throughout our lives. We need to get up and going *first thing in the morning*, challenge ourselves with a good exercise program early in the day, and then keep ourselves going—shopping, cleaning, watching grandkids, or volunteering for the remainder of the day. In this way, by the time we are ready for bed, we will be *good and tired*.

2. *Maintain your clock!*

Our clock is generally hardwired from birth, but it is entirely possible to disrupt our natural patterns and really mess up our sleep. One sure way to upset our clock is to expose our brains to "blue light" in the evening. Our brain sees blue light as *morning* and will wake back up! What is blue light? I am very sorry to say that TV and computers are both blue light. Ideally, we should not watch TV or use a computer after 6:00 p.m. so that we don't risk waking up our brains. On the other hand, getting bright light (such as being outside or using a light box) in the morning is an effective way to reenergize ourselves. Taking a brisk walk outside each morning is a great way to wake up our brains! In the evening hours, the use of a gentle yellow light, such as from a light bulb, is important to allow the brain to prepare for sleep. However, if your clock continues to be problematic and you are having trouble falling asleep in the evening, it *is* safe to use melatonin, 0.3 mg, in early evening. This safe medicine helps to adjust your clock to earlier evening hours so that you *can* fall asleep at 10:00 p.m. instead of 2:00 a.m.

3. *Manage your sleep trouble proactively!*

If, like Marcy's mom, worry creeps into the nighttime hours, I recommend keeping a pad of paper and pen next to the bed. When you go to bed, write down everything that is worrying you and everything you need to do the next day. If you wake in the night and are worried about something, *write it down* so that you can do it the next day. Often this helps to relieve anxiety and let your brain stop churning and finally fall asleep.

While I advise that we try to stay active, not obsess about a "bad night," and tell ourselves to relax so that the next night is better, sometimes these methods are just too hard to do. In this situation, I recommend *cognitive behavioral therapy* to help with sleep. Cognitive behavioral therapy, under the guidance of a trained psychologist or therapist, can assist you in making realistic changes to your sleep habits. It can help with sleep hygiene (explained below), assist in reducing negative sleep stimuli (e.g., worry at bedtime), and change negative perceptions about sleep—for example, I *must* have eight hours to feel rested! Excellent research evidence indicates that cognitive behavioral therapy is highly effective in improving sleep, and, what's more, it can often help with improving the rest of the day as well.

SO WHAT DO I DO IF I HAVE TO GET UP AND URINATE MULTIPLE TIMES EVERY NIGHT?

A majority of older men and some older women need to get up several times per night to urinate. Sometimes this is due to actual medical issues, such as an enlarged prostate or heart problems, but much of the time it is really a simple gravity problem. We all have blood vessels (veins) in our legs to move fluid back up from our legs to our kidneys so that we can urinate it out. These blood vessels have valves in them. As we age, these valves don't work as effectively as they used to, so when we are up on our feet all day long, excess liquid "pools" in our legs. At night, when we try to sleep, this fluid wakes us up, demanding to be excreted. But there are some things we can do to greatly help reduce the need for nighttime urination:

1. *Don't drink anything for three hours before bed.* Everyone should drink four to six eight-ounce glasses of fluid early in the day, but make sure you have drunk all this amount at least three hours before you want to go to sleep. Also avoid drinks with sugar in them.
2. *Prop your legs up higher than your heart* for thirty minutes before getting ready for bed.
3. *Don't drink alcohol or caffeine.* These are bladder irritants and often exacerbate urinary frequency.

Good "sleep hygiene" is essential to achieving a good night's rest. The following are the *top ten tips to sleeping well*:

1. *Keep a stable bedtime.*
2. *Keep the same awakening time.*
3. *Sleep only when you are sleepy. Don't force yourself to try to sleep.* Sleep only as much as you need to feel rested.
   - You should spend no more than twenty minutes lying in bed trying to fall asleep.
   - If you cannot fall asleep within twenty minutes, get up, go to another room, and read or find another relaxing activity until you feel sleepy again. Activities such as eating, balancing your checkbook, doing housework, watching TV, or studying for a test, which "reward" you for staying awake, should be avoided.
   - When you start to feel sleepy, you can return to bed. If you cannot fall asleep in another twenty minutes, repeat the process.
4. *If you must nap, take a nap for no longer than one hour and only in the afternoon.* Moreover, nap only in your bed. Remember, you want to associate the bed with sleepiness—not the sofa. If you cannot fall asleep within fifteen to twenty minutes, get out of bed. Nap only once each day. Try to nap at the same time of day. The best time is before 3:00 p.m.
5. *Avoid alcohol and caffeine entirely (including chocolate,* sorry!). Avoid heavy meals within four hours of bedtime. Avoid foods containing sugar.
6. *Do not smoke* (particularly in the evening).
7. *Don't go to bed hungry.*
8. *Reserve your bed for sleep* in a quiet, dark environment (no TV or radio on).
9. *Adopt a pre-bed routine* that might include a warm bath, reading, writing, or small snack.
10. *Adjust the bedroom environment* (light, noise, temperature) so that you are comfortable *before* you lie down.

LASTLY, WHAT ABOUT SLEEPING PILLS? CAN I USE THEM?

We would all like a pill that cures our problems—particularly our problems with sleep. Sleeping pills such as diphenhydramine (Benadryl, Tylenol PM, and many others), zolpidem (Ambien), lorazepam (Ativan), and many others are sold by the millions and do make people sleep longer, but they come with very high risk. These drugs have terrible side effects, especially for older people. They increase the danger of falling and risk of fracture, as well as augment confusion and cognitive decline. For someone like Marcy's mom, a sleeping pill that increased her risk of hip fracture could lead to a devastating outcome. She was given Trazodone, which is one of the "safer" medications for sleep, but even this routinely prescribed drug can cause low blood pressure and increased risk of confusion and should always be used with great caution. Rather than hoping to get a pill from a doctor to sedate you enough to sleep, I strongly encourage these other non-medication approaches to sleep management. They are highly effective, reduce the chance of perilous side effects, are far safer, and can help you to positively take charge of your life.

Good night!

· 37 ·

The Art of Caregiving

$\mathcal{T}$he true character of Vicki was buffered for a while longer because of one thing she did. She requested a change to her hours, asking to work a block of three days and nights rather than twelve-hour shifts. At the same time, Delores gave notice she was moving to another state in two months. That meant we had to find another caregiver—one who agreed to work four-day intervals at a stretch. By a stroke of good luck, Visiting Companions called to say that one of their best caregivers had just become available and would be able to accommodate that time slot.

And so, after a rough six months of questionable caregiving, providence at last kicked in. We met Helen the following week. Before her first day was over, we could tell Helen was smart, loyal, and highly experienced, and whereas Vicki kept telling us she had a heart but didn't, Helen really did have one.

The changes to my mother's healthcare and her overall well-being were subtle at first. But what became quickly visible was a revolution in my mother's attitude. Unlike days when Vicki was there and my mother spent most of her time comatose in her chair, when Helen was with her, I would go over and find my mother *singing*.

"As time goes by," my mom crooned happily as I entered, then continued humming a while longer. "I love the music Helen brings over," she chirped. "She knows *just* the songs I like!"

When I queried Helen, she admitted she had an extensive music library with hundreds of CDs.

"I like to find out what era of music a person resonates with," she explained. Then she went deeper. "We often forget that people who are in their eighties and nineties had good times. I like to discern what kind of music brings them joy. Even if the person can't 'tell' me, when they start to listen, there's usually some song that gets them actually singing along, with a brightness to their eyes. That's when I know I've hit upon something."

Before long I began seeing that Helen was a master at unlocking what made my mother tick. I suspected she had been like this with all her prior clients; that's why the families had loved her. Different from any caregiver I'd ever experienced and certainly unlike Vicki or Delores, Helen was a master sleuth with a mission to uncover clues to what had been satisfying memories to her clients. Once she discovered these, she built on them—which meant, for my mother, she added more and more articles of pleasure to her daily life.

For example, Helen discerned that my mother had traveled to Hawaii with my father. Were those fond memories? If yes, did she like the program *Hawaii 5-0*? Helen then rounded up videos of the old show, which my mother and she would watch together.

How about flowers? After a little detective work, Helen deduced that my mother was particularly fond of irises. Soon the two were on a "road trip" to tour the famed Schreiner's Iris Gardens, an hour from home. My mother loved it, and they each bought new varieties for their respective gardens. Helen planted my mother's bulbs in three spots in my mother's garden while my mother watched.

"They'll be beautiful next spring, Margaret," Helen said, giving my mother something to look forward to in the future.

That trip was such a success that Helen found out about other flower celebrations. Tulips were another favorite of my mother's. So when the Woodburn Tulip Festival opened, she took my mother—buying more bulbs that she planted in pots right outside the living room, where my mother would be able to see and enjoy them from her chair.

Next it *was* chairs. Which were my mother's favorites, and in what rooms? Helen was hunting for clues again, and it got my mother thinking. Before long an entirely new routine emerged. My mother's den had a comfortable chair, but more than that, the room faced east. It was lovely early in the day when the morning light poured in. That became her morning room. My mother's other favorite chair was in the living room. It was the chair that Elizabeth told her to *not* become too dependent on because it cheated her out of exercising her quadriceps. My mother loved it though—it had a button she could push that made it automatically rise up, boosting her to standing. But it was undeniably comfortable, and here she could rest in the afternoon and look out the window at the large, swaying Douglas fir trees off the patio. As the sun moved through the sky, it touched their needles with gold.

It was obvious that Helen was highly creative and something of an artist and interior decorator. Her brilliant idea of moving my mother from room to room to enjoy different scenery was like taking her on mini-vacations of the mind.

Reading poetry together was another breakthrough that provided immense delight. Helen soon had plumbed that my mother had been an English major and enjoyed literature. She also became aware that she had canoed the Yukon River several times with my father—at the ripe old age of seventy! Putting the two together, Helen asked one day whether she had ever heard of the poem "The Cremation of Sam McGee."

"I went to a small bar in Dawson City once and watched a man on a stage recite that poem," related Helen.

"I've been to that same bar and I know that poem!" said my mother, reliving another happy memory. Together they recited the poem out loud, which brought back a flood of recollections that she began describing to Helen about her adventures in the Yukon Territory.

When I later asked Helen how she knew that my mother would resonate with that poem, she admitted she didn't. It was just another attempt to excavate agreeable reminiscences of the past.

"I have a large collection of poetry books and also picture books for those who like to look at pictures. Even clients who have dementia love to look at paintings and photographs," she explained. "That's why I keep a library of books and music and movies from different times and different eras, and I try them all—hoping to find something that touches my person . . . that *means* something to them. And if my collection doesn't work, then I go to the library and keep trying until I do."

I thought about the time Helen invested and how it was making such a difference in my mother's daily life. The people Helen cared for weren't just patients; they were older individuals worthy of respect.

"It's different with everyone I've worked with," Helen went on. "But I truly believe that each person has something that brings them happy memories. And that's what I try to find—that *key to unlocking a happiness* for them."

When it came to my mother's actual healthcare regime, Helen rose to the top in that department too. In fact, she employed a uniquely new way of managing my mother's daily health schedule. She called it "continuity of care"—a term doctors used—and had developed what she termed "continuity sheets." Once she showed them to me, I immediately implemented them, seeing their value.

Continuity sheets were daily notations about everything pertaining to the people she cared for: what they ate; when they slept; what they did; what their mental status was; their energy level; their wants; their complaints. Documenting this each day on simple, straightforward charts she had designed made for an easy transition between caregivers. For example, if Vicki would write down what my mother had eaten for the past three days, Helen could make appropriate adjustments. If my mother had three days of prunes, Helen could deduce why she might be developing a slight case of diarrhea. To rectify that, Helen would lay off the prunes for a day. Or if all my mother had been served was meat each day, Helen shifted the diet to offer more vegetables.

Helen was very conscientious about diet.

The continuity sheets helped, too, with activities. If Vicki had had my mother out and about the day before, for instance, Helen would encourage my mother to stay home the next day and do restful activities, thereby keeping her energy levels up.

Beyond eating and outings, the continuity sheets kept track of potential problems. If my mother had been having trouble sleeping during Vicki's shift, Helen would be on the lookout for more confusion and respond accordingly. Further, it gave me a daily accounting of everything that went on concerning my mother when I wasn't there. Even more, the sheets provided an overview to anyone—including a healthcare professional or visiting nurse—the daily status of things.

After the continuity sheets were implemented (with a display of moaning and groaning from Vicki), I found my own peace of mind dramatically improved. I knew, from the sheets, that caregivers were really *observing*. Vicki was not happy and complained that Helen "cross-examined her" and that it "took time" to write down every day what my mom ate and whether she got constipated, but in this case I was firm. I insisted she comply. Vicki did, with reluctance.

In a few months' time, I began to see an even more drastic difference between Vicki and Helen's caregiving styles. Basically, there seemed to be a fundamental distinction in the way they approached their career. I suspected this was true among many of those who worked for older clients. For some, like Vicki, it was just a job. An employment where one could make a modest living in a tough job market. You didn't have to have much in the way of qualifications, education, or training. Vicki's bottom-line motivation, I was beginning to realize, was a paycheck.

But the incentive was entirely different for Helen—just as it had been for Inez and Alonzo. For caregivers such as these, the task was more than just another form of employment. It was, in fact, a ministry. Helen said it best one day, when I commented on her skill and kindness in taking care of my mother.

"I sure didn't grow up thinking 'I want to be a caregiver someday,' but I found out I loved it," she disclosed. "It was like I had found my calling and something that gave meaning to my life. You're going to laugh, but after my first experience taking care of a ninety-year-old client, I felt like it was God's hand in my life. It's like He said to me, 'This is what your career is going to be from now on, Helen Brooke.'"

She grinned, but I didn't laugh; I listened.

"You can't just feed old people and dress them, clean them up, and walk away," she continued. "There's no dignity for an older person in that. And that's what happens in nursing homes. I've seen it. There, old people lose touch with who they are; they forgo their individuality. Caregivers in centers often merely do what I refer to as 'feed, clean, and leave.' Even private caregivers do a disservice if they think that clamping their client in headphones and putting them in front of the TV and having them sit in a chair, hour after hour, is healthy. It's not healthy! It's the same thing as putting a toddler in front of a TV or computer screen all day to babysit them."

Helen shook her head. "What quality of life is that?"

Her words harked back to what I'd learned from journeying with my father through Alzheimer's disease. To have an existence of any worth, I had seen how vital it was for an old person to feel connected to people and to life, not segregated and apart from life.

"I believe it's part of a caregiver's responsibility to keep the one you are entrusted with *interested* in life; otherwise, you might as well put them in a cemetery," maintained Helen. "Make them feel they want to get up in the morning! But to do that you need to find out what they like . . . find out ways to keep them engaged! Plus, it makes the job more fun for you. I've had people try to tell me it's different if the patient has Alzheimer's. That's hogwash. I believe you can always find *something*, if you work at it, that will make a person happy."

My mother was listening to the conversation and smiling. Helen grinned back. "My duty as a caregiver is, of course, to keep your mom safe, clean, and fed," she said to both of us. "But it's also to help create a world to make Margaret happy."

And my mother was happy. She was especially satisfied at this moment because she was ready and dressed to go with Helen to do something that she enjoyed and that I refused to do with her because I hated it on principle: go to the casino and play the penny slot machines.

· 38 ·

Living to One Hundred

$\mathscr{F}$our days on, three days off. After close to a year of work, the differences in Vicki's and Helen's caregiving styles were effectively turning my weeks into boomerang trajectories. I quivered when Vicki was on, relaxed and rejoiced when it was Helen's turn. But I appeased my thinking by considering that when Helen was working, my mother had enough fun and attention to make up for all the other lower-quality days. And while I deliberated "retiring" Vicki, I knew that would be difficult: my mother had grown fond of her and felt, oddly, that she was doing Vicki a favor by employing her. Although it was backwards, she felt sympathy for Vicki and wanted to help her.

"Life's dealt Vicki so many cruel blows," expressed my mother, with concern. "She confided to me she had a terrible relationship with her mother; they fought continually, and her mother never understood her. Her mother's been dead for ten years, and Vicki still feels bad they never reconciled."

My mother looked thoughtful. "She's told me that I am the mother she'd always hoped for, and she's asked me to stand in, in her mother's place, at her wedding."

"That still doesn't make up for the fact that Vicki dropped the garage door on your mom's head and another time walked away from her at the curb, when your mom fell because she couldn't see it," John commented to me, remaining skeptical of Vicki. "I worry you are making a mistake keeping her, Mar. On Vicki's watch, your mother has had to have two CT scans."

Undeniably, my mother had been fortunate both times that she hadn't broken anything nor suffered hemorrhagic concussions. But after talking it over with Visiting Companions, they said they were actively training Vicki. As well, after each mishap Vicki was verbally contrite. Even more, it was my mother who always wanted to give Vicki one more chance.

"It's not her fault; it's because she's had so much instability in her life," my mother reasoned. "And that's why Lennie is so good for her. He's a stabilizing influence. I think I am, too, for her. Vicki does have such a compassionate heart, and she loves me. I can't disappoint her by letting her go."

With my mother's ninetieth birthday coming up, though, Vicki said she didn't want to be any part of it.

"In my experience, it's better to just let these days pass on by unnoticed," Vicki said.

Like so many of her statements, I wondered what in her past had brought her to this sour conclusion. Helen, however, was delighted over the celebration and between her, my mother, and me, we drew up a guest list. There was a surprise element, too: my mother wasn't privy to the information that my sisters were going to fly in from out of town and both Emily and Jennifer would travel home from college for it. Everyone was excited for September 27—that is, except for Vicki. As we neared the big day, I reiterated that she and Lennie were, of course, invited.

"We'll show up," Vicki said, with characteristic pessimism. "The reason I think it's a mistake to make a big deal is because of what happened on my own grandmother's ninetieth birthday."

I didn't care to hear more, but she ran on anyway.

"My grandma was kind of a crank. My mom planned a birthday party for her, even though Grandma didn't want it. She said she'd rather die than have a party thrown for her. Well, my mom was just as stubborn and she did it anyway. Right after the party, my grandma said she needed to lie down. An hour later, when my mom went to check on her, she found her *dead*."

The party was a grand success, though, and my mother enjoyed herself immensely. Vicki did not attend, citing a headache, but everyone else came, much to my mother's delight. She was thrilled having everyone home, and she had looked beautiful. Tina had done her hair; Helen had applied makeup and helped her select her pretty black St. John suit with the gold piping to wear. Throughout the evening, my mother sparkled, looking at least a decade younger than her age. Surrounded by all those who loved her and feeling well, she expressed that perhaps, after all, she just might choose to live to be one hundred.

Two weeks later there was more good news. When seeing Dr. Thompson at an early-morning appointment for her annual physical, the physician was pleased with her progress.

"You are indeed more frail than a year ago, Margaret, and I want you to make sure you use your walker all the time now and continue to exercise," she commented. "But you have a good bill of health and," she said, smiling, "are also *as strong as a horse*."

"Darn," said my mother when she got back in the car, appearing distressed.

"What's wrong?"

"Well, since Dr. Thompson said I must use my walker all the time now, that means I can't go running with you anymore."

I laughed. She never lost her sense of humor.

"I will never understand what joy you get out of jogging," she added, attaching her seatbelt. "And Daddy liked it too and put all those old patients in running shoes."

I brought her to her home to rest for a few hours and went back to work. After such a fine physical, I said I would return at one o'clock to take her out to lunch to celebrate. I asked Vicki to make sure my mom put on the same black suit—the one she loved and had worn at her birthday party—for this was to be a special occasion.

Just as I was wrapping up a bit of writing, my cell phone rang. I saw it was Vicki—probably calling with a question about clothes or to say they were running a little late. But Vicki wasn't calling to talk about clothes. Instead, her voice was strangely cool.

"I need to know what you want me to do," she mumbled dully. "You see, there's been an accident."

• *39* •

And They Shall Inherit the Earth

"*I* didn't know she was going to stand up," Vicki justified.

I felt a chill to my innermost bones. "What happened, Vicki?"

She took a breath. "Your mom fell down the stairs."

Still speaking in a monotone, Vicki admitted she hadn't attached the seat belt and let my mother push the button to move the stairglide herself. She said she walked away "just for a second" toward the garage, not realizing that the chair had stopped five steps up from the bottom. My mother, not able to see but thinking she was at the ground floor, stood up and took a step. She now lay on the hard tile floor, unmoving.

The blood coursing in my body froze in my veins. "Is she alive, Vicki?"

"She's breathing but unconscious. She landed on her face," Vicki replied as detachedly as if she were talking about a glass that had spilled.

"Why didn't you belt her in!"

"I forgot. Should I wait for you to come over?"

I could hardly control my emotions. Vicki was an idiot. "Call 911. And do not move her! We don't know the condition of her neck. Have the paramedics call me immediately on my cell; I am leaving for the hospital now. It will take me thirty minutes. You should get there in fifteen. I will see you there."

The ambulance driver phoned in less than ten minutes. He asked specific questions and said that the "black-headed lady" had given him a sheet with my mother's medical history and prescriptions—the health form I had made and put up on the refrigerator. He said they were treating her injuries as if she had a broken neck and other broken bones. She was bleeding quite heavily from her forehead. She remained unconscious.

The interminable drive to the hospital gave me ample time to reflect on my utter stupidity in keeping Vicki on, just because my mother felt sorry for her. This was all my fault! John had been right from the beginning: in a case of caregivers, *one strike, you're out*! Never again would I make that mistake. If she survived, never again would I make allowances for lack of judgment or character. The price tag was enormously too high.

My mother was already being seen in the emergency department when I arrived. Entering her examining room, I thought at first I must have made a mistake: this could not be a person I knew. Only from the bloodied black suit lying crumpled on a swivel chair could I have guessed I was in the right place.

My mother's face was swollen grotesquely. Large, concentric circles of bruised flesh surrounded her eye bones, giving the appearance of a raccoon. Her tissue-paper skin, from her brows to her jaw, revealed internal bleeding from blood already thinned by Coumadin. The flesh of her face was a mask of purple and mottled brown, while the bandage wrapping her forehead oozed bright red with fresh blood.

"We have multiple things going on," said the ER doctor solemnly upon entering, "and are going to run a number of tests. Most importantly, we want to make certain that her neck isn't broken and do a CT scan to see whether she has any significant bleeding in her brain."

He gave me a moment to let his words sink in as he perused the health history sheet I'd made. "This is very helpful. Did you write this?"

"Yes, with the help of my mother's geriatrician, Dr. Thompson."

"I will let Dr. Thompson know about your mother. We're also going to image her back, ribs, pelvis, and legs for fractures and run blood work. When we get some results, I'll be back."

Shaking, I picked up my mother's skirt from the chair and sat down, placing the clothes on my lap. Dazedly, I fingered them while staring at my mother's beleaguered body. How could this possibly be the same woman who was laughing and smiling only a few hours ago?

By the time a medley of tests and labs were run, John had joined me and now sat, unbelieving, by my side. Wondering where Vicki was, I tried calling her several times but got no answer. I also left a message for Helen to tell her the unhappy news.

The assessments, when they came back bit by bit, were both good and bad. The positive news was that my mother's neck was not broken—in fact, she had not sustained any broken bones except for a few cracked ribs, which was nothing short of a miracle. And while she had suffered a concussion, she was not, at this point, exhibiting dangerous bleeding on the brain. Her labs showed a urinary tract infection, which I actually considered good news, as I presumed it was easily treatable. My mother was to be hospitalized for observation (she was still unconscious) and for subsequent tests.

I relayed the information to Emily and Jennifer and my sisters—all of whom were debating rushing home. After some discussion, we decided that everyone should wait before reacting . . . we would know more after Dr. Thompson arrived and Nana had "come to."

"But what if she doesn't wake up?" said Jennifer anxiously.

Both Emily and Jennifer decided to drive home from college to see their beloved grandmother.

At eight o'clock I called Vicki again, finding it strange that she had not returned any of my voice messages nor arrived at the hospital. An hour later, I was startled to see Helen standing at the door, carrying a small satchel.

"I wanted to give you a break so you could go home and rest tonight." She lifted her bag. "I came prepared." She then glanced at my mother. "Oh my God. Oh, Margaret!"

John ushered Helen inside. I appreciated her concern and wondered again about Vicki, and I asked Helen whether she might know what happened to her. "She seems to have vanished from the face of the earth."

"In a way," answered Helen, "she has. She didn't tell you?"

"Tell me what?"

"Vicki's got a new job. I didn't know until this afternoon either. She won't be coming back."

"*What?*"

"Evidently, it's been in the works for some time. Two weeks ago, Visiting Companions found her a new position. Apparently, she's starting with the client tomorrow."

"You're kidding," I said, dumbstruck. "No two-week notice? Just abandoning my mother?"

"Yes, that's a good word for it." Helen plopped her suitcase on the floor. "So this afternoon, I quit too! Not your mother, but Visiting Companions. They admitted they acted unethically. But I guess Vicki was pushing and pushing them for it. They assured me they're trying to find another caregiver for your mom. I think you'd be better off without them, however."

In my mind, Visiting Companions—and everyone connected with them, aside from Helen—was unilaterally *fired*. I would never deal with them again.

"I wonder whether Vicki's new client would be so anxious to have her if they could see her old client," said John angrily, motioning to my prostrate mother.

"You were right about her mean eye," I muttered miserably.

"Don't blame yourself, Mar," John said adamantly.

"He's right. Vicki had even me fooled," offered Helen. "We'll be more careful next time."

If there was a next time, I thought, with a sinking heart.

By the next morning my mother had opened her eyes a few times but had still not uttered a word. Helen, who slept in the chair next to my mother's bed, said she'd had a few "run-ins" with the shift nurses. One had told her she couldn't stay in the same room and would have to sleep down the hall—the same lounge I had been forced into during my mother's TIA. Helen flatly refused. The nurse argued. Helen stayed firm. The nurse lost the battle.

But the other nurses Helen dealt with nearly gave her a coronary.

"*This* is why I don't like the hospital," she spouted, still agitated. "Two out of three times, I had to tell the nurse or aide to wash her hands! I don't care if someone says they used the disinfectant *in the hallway*. That's not good enough. I tell them I want them to wash their hands *in the sink, with soap*, before they change your mom's IVs or catheter."

Helen could be a guard dog, standing her ground. And she was exactly what my mother needed.

"But what really riles me is that just before you got here, an aide tried to draw a urine sample from out of your mom's catheter," she continued. "But she took it out of the wrong port, deflated the internal balloon, and the suprapubic catheter came out! When I pointed out what she had done, she went out to get another nurse. That one apologized, took another sample, and replaced the catheter. I'm not a nurse, but that's a surefire recipe for infection."

Helen was obviously tired, but she would never admit it. "I'm going to get a coffee and then be back," she said. "They don't give you anything to drink here, either, except for the scant half-pint juice that comes on the tray. No wonder your mom has to stay on IV fluids. I feel like I'm in the Sahara, with nothing to drink."

Hospitals were also poorly lit, I thought, judging from the lighting of the room. Right now, the fluorescent glow made my mother's black and blue face and arms appear even worse. The room's tiny window faced a brick wall and let in no healing sunlight. And it was noisy. It sounded to me like all the pagers and beepers of the hospital must be going off at once, and the hard linoleum floor surface only magnified the acoustics.

Maybe it was not a bad thing my mother was only semiconscious. There would be no rest for her here.

When Dr. Thompson arrived, she said that my mother's current set of labs was showing that her bladder infection was caused by enterococci and pseudomonas bacteria. From her expression, as well as from some reading I had done, I knew enough to understand that was not good. Those bugs were among the super bad guys.

"We don't want your mother to go septic—meaning, have these bacteria escape to her blood stream," said Dr. Thompson, gravely. "I have ordered the antibiotic vancomycin for her, to be given intravenously."

"What happens if they do get into her blood?" asked Helen.

"Then the condition changes dramatically."

The question I wanted to ask, but was too cowardly, was: Did her compromised state resulting from her trauma affect her resistance? When you were weak and frail to begin with, then got an infection, and then on top of that suffered an injury, making you even weaker and more frail, was your immune system up to the task of stemming the tide of a super bug?

In an indirect way, Dr. Thompson answered the question without my even posing it. "Since Margaret has come into the hospital, she has developed some atelectasis in the lower left lobe of her lung. I want to keep a watch on it and have a chest x-ray done to see whether it's early pneumonia," said Dr. Thompson.

"Is it from the accident?" I queried.

"The accident isn't helping matters," replied the doctor.

For the next three days, my mother was given the "big gun" antibiotic, but while I prayed for improvement, subsequent lab work came back showing the opposite. The dangerous bacteria were not being eradicated. Rather, they were continuing to multiply. The vancomycin was not effective.

"I was hoping this would not be the case," said Dr. Thompson, pondering. "How are you feeling, Margaret?"

My mother merely mumbled. Since the fall, she had uttered only a few incoherent sentences. "This is an unfortunate scenario," added the doctor, with her eyes still on my mother's frail form. "I am going to have the hospital infectious disease specialist weigh in with his opinion on this."

I sighed, knowing *exactly* what the infectious disease specialist would say—because he had said it before. When my mother was presumably dying two years ago, he had told Dr. Hip that he would not treat her. In fact, Dr. Hip had relayed his comments during one of our final conversations before my mother was moved to Soothing Breezes. The words now came back to me with a vengeance:

"The super bugs will win in the end," the specialist had said. "In the end, the bugs will take over the earth."

· *40* ·

Go *GICU!* Stop *Step-Down!*

*A*s I expected, a few days later the antibiotic was stopped. The doctor signing the order was the infectious diseases specialist. In a fit of desperation, when I queried Dr. Thompson about it, she reiterated that the drug was not reducing the spread of the dangerous bacteria embattling my mother's weak body. She explained that the specialist felt, with the failure of vancomycin— arguably the most potent weapon in a doctor's arsenal against super bug infections—nothing more could be done for my mother. In his opinion, it was now only a matter of time.

Dr. Thompson listened once more to my mother's congested lungs and stared contemplatively at her pummeled face. An accompanying geriatric nurse stood on the other side of the bed.

"So what can we do?" I asked, feeling heartbroken. "Anything?"

Dr. Thompson didn't respond. Passing in front of me as if I had ceased to exist, she walked out of the room, stopping on the other side of the door, and crossed her arms. The nurse motioned for me to remain still.

"She does this," she said, quietly. "Just wait. She's thinking."

Something about the physician's posture was riveting. From the intense look of concentration on her face, it seemed that the earth must have just stopped revolving. The minutes ticked by, and still Dr. Thompson didn't move. This did not seem the attitude of someone who had given up and moved on. Rather, she was taking time to distill disparate complexities of an elderly patient presenting multiple problems interfacing and compounding one another.

At that moment I saw clearly that the greatest physicians called upon the healing properties of three things: science, art, and empathy. Dr. Thompson was digging deeply in her professional medical bag and broad experience in the field of geriatrics, searching for answers. Observing her gave me a hope I was trying to deaden.

When she came back into the room, her mind seemed to be made up.

"We are on a tightrope," Dr. Thompson stated deliberately, "and I am going to try one last thing. Whether it works or not remains to be seen. I am prescribing a PICC line to be put in today for your mother. Also, I am moving her to a new room."

She turned her gaze to speak directly to my mother, whose eyes had fluttered open.

"And Margaret, I am making you a cocktail."

This cocktail was not one's normal libation, and it didn't come in a highball glass. Rather, it was something Dr. Thompson formulated, acting like an artisan brewmaster. She blended a combination of three antibiotics—vancomycin, gentamicin, and ceftazidime—to be dosed through my mother's PICC line, like a rebel artillery sent to try to defeat the giant army of enterococci and pseudomonas bacteria whose mission was to kill my mother.

That was Dr. Thompson's primary strategy. But she had other lines of attack as well. When taken together, they were, in effect, a hospital makeover.

When Dr. Thompson said she wished my mother moved to another room, she was not merely transferring her to another space down the hall. She had my mother moved to a room much larger and one that had a window that looked out upon, not a wall of brick, but the sky and trees and afternoon sunshine. She explained that my mother should have every advantage possible to offset sensory impairment at the hospital. For example, she needed better lighting. Knowing that my mother had macular degeneration, Dr. Thompson said that good lighting was imperative to her sense of well-being. She asked us to make sure her hearing aid was operating and had us get fresh batteries. She removed the oxygen lines from her nose, saying my mother's oxygen levels were ample and the lines connecting to the tank acted like a tether. Same thing for IV fluids and IV antibiotics. All of them were just more leashes, and now that she had a PICC line, my mother could have infusions at scheduled intervals and didn't need to be restrained by an IV stand all day.

As much as my mother hurt to move, Dr. Thompson requested that she attempt to. Bed rest equaled muscle wasting—a dangerous complication possible to anyone confined in a hospital, but especially older persons. To achieve the goal of increasing mobility, she told the nurses and us to get my mother up and out of bed as much as my mother could tolerate. With the oversight from a physical therapist, my mother was to endeavor to transfer several times a day from her bed to a chair. And, as her strength improved, she was to try walking a few steps with her walker, under surveillance, of course. All of these things increased her chances of regaining a modicum of her prior independence.

Finally, Dr. Thompson was concerned about my mother developing delirium. To offset the possibility, she hoped to keep her biological clock—her days and nights—as normal as possible. Nurses on the unit had already been informed that they were *not* to wake up my mother during the night hours. Dosing, procedures, vital sign readings were to occur before 11:00 p.m. and after 6:30 a.m. That meant no more changing catheters at 1:00 a.m. or 3:00 a.m. blood draws. My mother's ability to sleep in the hospital, Dr. Thompson reiterated, was critical to keep her from developing a *hospitalization-associated disability* and stepping down permanently.

It was a term I had never heard before.

"These are step-downs that occur after hospitalization and are not related to what brought the patient to the hospital in the first place," Dr. Thompson took the time to explain. "Many times, patients are living independently before the episode, but when they leave the hospital, they can't do so any longer. Older patients get weak from too much bed rest. They lose a sense of their days and nights. They suffer sleep deprivation. They are overly medicated. They get more and more confused and fall into delirium. Hospitalization-associated disabilities happen to over half of all the older patients we currently treat in the hospital. Although we can treat what they were admitted for—such as a urinary tract infection or pneumonia—most of them at discharge will have lost their ability to be independent. In fact, their poor prognosis is the same as for older individuals hospitalized for hip fracture."

Doing the math, I remembered my dad had died only eleven months after fracturing his hip. "So what can we do?" I asked, feeling slightly terrified, not only for old people but for when my turn came.

"There are steps that can reduce or even prevent this disability from happening. But it's going to require changes. The best intervention is what is being done at a few hospitals around the country. Implementing geriatric inpatient units, or, as we call them, "ACE," or acute care or elder units. These places are different. They are structured to try to minimize deconditioning. It's a geriatric team approach."

She motioned to my mother. "You've seen some of the techniques I'm implementing for your mother. Reducing drugs. Keeping track of a patient's baseline—especially when they enter the hospital. Getting patients moving. Allowing them to sleep at night. Making things look and feel more like home and less like the hospital. Having touchstones to keep patients *oriented*. We don't have the luxury in Oregon of having any geriatric care units yet."

I was dying to know more, but Dr. Thompson was paged. "Your mother's bacteria count is going down," she said, departing for the next patient. "I think the new therapy is showing signs of effectiveness."

My heart danced with the good news, yet Dr. Thompson left me with lots to think about. Life when you're old, as the neurologist had said years before, was a roller coaster ride! For my mother and father, one minute they were well, the next they were sick. Then they were well again—but maybe not quite at the same level. As I had observed, so much could impact how far they came back. It was more than just a factor of their own basic health or genes, but so much depended on things that happened *outside them*—like hospital stays or doctors or healthcare officials who truly understood old people and age-related diseases and issues—or not. Those factors indeed could influence the difference between life and death. Or, if not that extreme, at least how much quality of life remained for a senior citizen.

Geriatric inpatient care units. I tossed the notion around in my mind. It was a fascinating concept. I knew, from having a doctor for a father who spent most of his life working in hospitals, that many hospitals had "NICUs"—neonatal intensive care units—and "PICUs"—pediatric intensive care units. It made perfect sense, I thought, that hospitals should also offer something strictly for older patients, especially if such a unit could keep them from having to suffer steep declines or, as Dr. Thompson said, "step-downs" from hospitalization-associated disabilities.

In my mind, I came up with the perfect term.

GICU.

GICU (sounding like "gick you"), standing for *geriatric inpatient care unit*. In my mind's eye, I could already visualize a bumper sticker emblazoning an AARP member's auto:

"Go GICU! Stop Step-Down!"

It made absolute sense. A GICU with specialized geriatric teams headed by geriatricians like Dr. Thompson could make a positive difference in so many people's lives. And mine too—when I got there.

I glanced again at my mother, feeling a powerful rush of gratitude. After a week, some of the black around her eyes was turning yellow, and the heavy swelling in her face was reducing enough so that her oval face, which had been so pretty, was beginning to show a resemblance to who she was eight days ago. She was going to survive—thanks to a phenomenal geriatrician who had fought for her and a revolutionary new way of administering hospital care. My mother had dodged another bullet, and we were blessed.

The scary thing, I thought, was that in today's reality, too many old people would never have a geriatrician, or a GICU, or live long enough to know the critical difference both could make in their healthcare outcome.

What I Wish I'd Known

The Serious Problems of Today's Hospitals for Older Adults—Why We Need to Demand a Change *Now*

Elizabeth Eckstrom, MD, MPH, MACP

*O*lder adults are a unique group when it comes to being admitted to a hospital. Their needs, reactions, and future prognoses are entirely different from those of middle-aged persons. Unfortunately, many hospitals today are not set up well to attend to the special concerns of older persons. This lack of understanding of the aging patient's specialized requirements results in management that can actually harm them and dramatically affect the life they will lead after leaving the hospital.

Many people go to the hospital for a major medical illness or event, such as a heart attack, hip fracture, or pneumonia. Hospital teams are well equipped to attend to these problems. They know how to care for your heart, give you a new hip, or treat your pneumonia. For elderly persons, the problem is often not the disease that brought them to the hospital in the first place; it is *what happens to them when they are in the hospital.*

Many of them will develop what is termed a "hospital-associated disability." This is functional decline that occurs between the onset of the acute illness and discharge from the hospital. Even when the illness that necessitated them being in the hospital is "cured," one out of three patients aged seventy and older will leave the hospital functionally worse off. *This major "step-down" is often permanent.*

The usual scenario is this: an older person who lives independently develops an illness that brings him to the hospital. He is treated for that condition and then discharged. But upon leaving the hospital, that same patient will have acquired a major new disability that wasn't present before, such as trouble walking or memory problems. No longer is he able to live independently. He has lost the ability to manage what geriatricians call the ADLs, or activities of daily living—or being able to walk, bathe, dress, or use the toilet without assistance. From then on, the patient will need the help of caregivers or require long-term care.

In short, "hospital-associated disabilities" are downhill spirals. A critical risk factor is your age. The older you are, the more likely it is you will leave the hospital disabled. And among patients who acquire a disability, less than half will ever recover to their pre-illness level of functioning. Nursing home placement and death rates are high.

Hospital-associated disabilities fall into six major categories: (1) confusion and delirium, (2) urination problems, (3) constipation and bowel issues, (4) weakness, (5) skin breakdown, and (6) functional decline. What are these, and how can you protect yourself and your loved ones from developing them? Even more, how can hospital protocols be changed to minimize the chances of older patients developing them?

1. *Confusion, delirium, and cognitive impairment* commonly occur when older patients are in the hospital. Both of Marcy's parents experienced brain problems. Research reveals that as many as 40 percent of older people leave the hospital with cognitive impairment or worsened memory. While many gradually return to their prior baseline over several weeks or months, others do not. They may not remember instructions given to them at discharge, or they may have trouble taking pills or doing things easily managed before they went into the hospital. It is essential, therefore, to try to minimize cognitive problems during a hospital stay.

There are several ways to do this. Be sure to frequently *orient* parents or loved ones while they are in the hospital so that they are aware of where they are. Have them maximize their use of hearing aids and eyeglasses. Work to optimize their sleep. Keep them as mobile as possible during their hospital stay. And strive to minimize medications that worsen brain function.

As previously mentioned, many doctors have little training in polypharmacy and can accidentally prescribe wrong medications to older persons. Ask the doctor questions about *each medication* being prescribed to an older patient. Also feel free to request to talk with the pharmacist—a key player—to be sure your loved one is not getting something that could worsen confusion. ***See Appendix 1 (the Beers List) and print it out.*** This documents the most dangerous drugs for older people. If your loved one is admitted to the hospital and prescribed one of the drugs on the list, speak with the hospital team to see whether the medication could be avoided or there is a safer choice.

2. *Urination* can easily become problematic when older individuals are hospitalized. First, if they are very sick, they may receive a Foley catheter—a tube that goes directly into their bladder and allows urine to flow into a bag worn outside the body. This prevents patients from needing to get up to go to the bathroom. While sounding convenient (and at times it *is* essential for care), often catheters are not necessary and cause trouble. Catheters increase the risk of urinary tract infections as well as the potential for urinary retention once they are removed. Marcy's mother had ongoing problems with her catheter.

It is far better to have the nursing staff assist an older, hospitalized patient to the bathroom on a regular basis—approximately every two hours during the day—or to help them use a bedside commode. This prevents the need for inserting a catheter and greatly reduces the risk for complications. Keep in mind, though, it is usually *not* a good idea to leave timing of urination up to older patients. If they wait until they feel the need to go and push the button for the nurse, it may be a long wait for the nurse to come assist them. Often by this time they have had an accident and are miserable. *Timed voiding*, or assisting a person to the bathroom regularly, is therefore important to prevent this from happening.

3. Constipation is another hospital danger that most people don't think of. Immobility, often as a result of medical illness, can lead to uncomfortable constipation. Dehydration, a common occurrence when people are sick, as well as new medications, especially pain pills, and even such things as a bland hospital diet and a different environment can all contribute to poorly functioning bowels. Beyond discomfort, constipation can lead to urinary retention and urinary tract infection, confusion, decreased appetite, and rectal pain and bleeding. It is worthwhile to talk with the nurses about keeping your loved one's bowels regular. If your parent needs something to treat constipation, MiraLAX (polyethylene glycol) has been shown to be safe and effective for many older adults. Milk of magnesia, however, can be highly dangerous in older persons with kidney problems and should be avoided in most older individuals.

4. Weakness is a peril of hospitalization. Each day an older patient is in the hospital and on bed rest, it takes a minimum of *two days* afterward to regain his strength. There are three main reasons for this. First, for a patient on bed rest, not as much oxygen is going to the muscles. Second, unused muscles become stiffer and smaller. Third, lung function rapidly declines as each day passes. Many older people, of course, have a reason they are inactive; they may have just had a heart attack or are suffering with severe pneumonia, for example. Nevertheless, it is essential that a physical therapist see them expeditiously to determine whether there are bed exercises they can do and to be sure the patient is getting up and moving *as soon as possible.*

Sometimes patients are immobilized and kept in bed because they are attached to tubes (IV tubes, Foley tubes, heart monitors, etc.). If this is the case, it is essential to get the tubes out, at least for a while, so that they can get out of bed and be as active as they are able.

5. *Skin issues* are particularly troublesome when older people are hospitalized. The aging skin is at high risk of breakdown and pressure ulcers; this threat increases with each day for an elderly patient in the hospital. Why? When in the hospital, older persons usually move around very little, often have poor nutrition (not caring to eat hospital food), and may have less-than-ideal attention to episodes of urinary or bowel incontinence. It is therefore critical each day your loved one is in the hospital that a nursing team assesses him or her for skin issues. To prevent dangerous and painful skin breakdown in aging patients, nurses must encourage ambulation, turn older persons frequently if they truly cannot get up, ensure they are receiving adequate nutrition, and be highly conscientious of bowel and bladder care. Marcy asked Helen, her mother's caregiver, to perform this while Margaret was in the hospital.

6. *Functional decline,* or the loss of aspects of independent living, routinely affect older people in the hospital. In fact, statistics show that more than 50 percent of adults older than eighty-five will leave the hospital with a major new disability, rendering them unable to perform the same level of self-care they did before they entered. *These "step-downs" are not inevitable and can often be prevented.* Yet it takes vigilance to keep them from occurring. Having patients remain active and engaged, well-oriented, and eating and sleeping well is vital to prevent decline.

Some hospitals in the United States have developed an exceptional program to reduce the occurrence of hospital-associated disabilities among older persons. Called *"Acute Care of the Elderly"* or ACE units, these specialized units consist of multidisciplinary teams with expertise in older adults. The units themselves have significant environmental modifications.

The ACE unit team is composed of a geriatrician, nurses, physical and occupational therapists, social workers, dietitians, and other geriatrics experts who work together comprehensively. This fully integrated approach has been shown to be more effective than when consultation services are performed in isolation. Together, the team provides oversight and geriatric assessment, beginning at *admission to the hospital.*

Evaluation of an older person's level of function upon entering the hospital is essential to optimize their function when discharged. When your parent or loved one is admitted, make sure the doctor in charge documents your parent's *baseline before the onset of the illness or incident*. What activities of daily living could she perform? Could she bathe or take a shower by herself? Take her own medications? What equipment does she use for walking—a cane? A walker? What is her level of cognition? Often, a family member or caregiver needs to relay this information. **For an excellent template for a *health history sheet*, see Appendix 2.** In this way it is possible to assess the level of functional decline that may be occurring from the hospital stay and not from the acute illness itself.

In many hospitals, the nursing team gathers information about function, but it doesn't get communicated to the doctors. Marcy can testify to that! In fact, more than 50 percent of the time, functional status is not considered by the physician team. Additionally, core measurements of cognition and ADLs should be assessed in daily rounds as well.

ACE units are reengineered to meet the needs of older patients. Often, they have carpeted floors to increase and encourage ambulation. Interventions to mitigate loud, disorienting noises are employed. Patients who are able to bathe or dress themselves are encouraged to do so and even to dress in their street clothing instead of hospital gowns. Family members are encouraged to stay with patients overnight. Processes that restrict mobility, such as orders for excessive bed rest, are avoided. Protocols are put in place to promote sleep (keep a patient to a day/night schedule), promote hydration, and make sure that aids for sensory impairment are used. Some ACE units also advise bringing meals from home to help keep an older person eating and oriented. Lastly, some studies have shown that natural beauty—through patient room windows and exposure to nature—can have significant healing properties.

These new geriatric interdisciplinary care units—that Marcy termed "GICU"—have been shown to reduce the incidence of functional decline at discharge. Plus, studies show an increased likelihood that the patient who had been independent can be *discharged to home*! ACE units reduce hospital length of stay and result in cost savings. At the same time, they offer increased satisfaction among patients, their families, and their physicians!

Hospital-associated disabilities have a terribly high price tag attached—financially and emotionally—and the stakes are high. Specialized changes can make for profoundly different and optimistic results. Hopefully, ACE teams will become standard practice at all our hospitals to ensure that the needs of older adults are attended to . . . along with the heart attacks and fractures that originally brought them into the hospital.

As Marcy says, *"Go GICU!"*

No More Dresses

$\mathcal{My}$ mother pulled through. More than that, she was able to go home.

None of us ever saw, or heard, from Vicki again. It continued to shock me that she had never even bothered to call to see if my mother had lived or died. From then on, I had a perpetual chill whenever I read about caregivers who—through ineptitude or design—took advantage of, or harmed, their older clients. Helen said, in her opinion, if a nursing home or caregiver refused to allow a camera to be put up in a client's room, there was something they wanted to hide.

Camera or not, we had come perilously close to the edge. After my mother's discharge from the hospital, I joined the ranks of patient families who referred to Dr. Thompson as "The Miracle Worker." She had saved my mother's life.

At last, for a glorious time, there was peace. We were fortunate to find a new caregiver to pair with Helen—one who met our new, stiff requirements. Life settled into a calmer routine, with space to breathe again, and a sense that maybe there was some predictability to life after all. We enjoyed more birthdays and festive celebrations together and began to forget (well, not exactly—but the outlines were dimmer) what the ER looked like during the holidays.

As the weeks went by, my mother's swelling and bruises began to greatly diminish, although she would always have a dent in her forehead. But the terrible green and purple "prizefighter" countenance could now be concealed with a little makeup. She regained her interest in life—going out to lunch, listening to books on tape, and visiting gardens with Helen.

There was a difference though. The latest episode had taken a toll on my mother's overall endurance, and she had lost some of the resiliency she once had when facing any infection.

Like many women, and men too, my mother succumbed to recurrent urinary tract infections, or UTI's, as she got older. After the accident, they seemed to be increasingly frequent, and were more troublesome, much to my mother's dismay.

Before long, we came to know the symptoms—indications commonly observed in older persons—urinary frequency, pain, confusion, and weakness. Dr. Thompson became concerned, as we all were, about why my mother was so susceptible to repeated urinary tract infections. Each one seemed to leave her slightly more frail. She suggested we consult an urologist, Dr. Kemper, to gain his professional perspective. My mother was keen to do it, hoping to stave off more "episodes"—the word she had learned to despise, when referring to her UTI's.

Dr. Kemper conducted a thorough evaluation. The results revealed something none of us had ever known about my mother, including herself. She had a congenital abnormality of her right ureter—probably since birth —but for the past ninety years it had never been a problem. Now, though, it was acting up. And there was not just one ureter on her right side, she actually had two: duplicated ureters coming from her bladder. One had become diseased, with two obstructions.

This was keeping her bladder from emptying, contributing to the infections.

Dr. Kemper concluded that, considering her advanced age, the best treatment was to insert something called a "supra-pubic catheter" into her bladder, which could work to bypass the malfunctioning ureter and keep her bladder drained.

My mother, understandably, was concerned. "What's that? Does it require surgery?" she asked. From her previous experience at the hospital, I knew she was desperate to stay away as long as possible.

"Yes it does," Dr. Kemper answered gently. "A supra-pubic catheter is a sterile, flexible tube, like a tiny garden hose. I would put it directly into your bladder through an incision in your belly just above your pelvic bone. Its purpose is to drain urine before it can accumulate and start another infection. The tubing attaches to a collecting bag that you would wear outside of your body."

My mother looked shocked, then deflated. "Like a colostomy bag?"

"Sort of," said Dr. Kemper, slowly, "but really, people get used to it before long. During the day, you can wear a smaller storage bag that straps on your leg and can be concealed. At night, we recommend you wear the larger bag, and attach it to your bed."

"If she doesn't have the surgery?" I asked.

"In your mother's case, that's a poor option," said Dr. Kemper. "She would continue succumbing to infections that eventually would destroy her kidney, and likely result in sepsis."

Later, Dr. Thompson set my mother's mind a bit more at ease. "The surgery is not a difficult one," she explained. "And, Margaret, the procedure is not what I would call 'extraordinary measures.' I know you do not want that. While an indwelling catheter and collecting bag does create inconvenience, thousands of people do well with this approach."

My mother, without too much deliberation, decided upon surgery. As Dr. Thompson said, it was not extreme, and required only one night in the hospital. Helen stayed with her. The following morning I was happy to find my mother in good spirits, well oriented, and with minimal pain.

She noticed my glance at the collecting bag hanging by a hook on a low rail of the hospital bed. She shook her head. "I'll just have to get used to this thing."

"If it keeps you well for several more years, it's worth it," I said, meaning it with all my heart.

Transitioning to live with a new, tethering accessory was not easy, however. It required a whole new routine which took time and careful maintenance. Getting used to the ordeal increased my mother's daily fatigue. She rested for longer periods in her chair and felt awkward going out to do some of the things she usually did, and those activities seemed to make her more tired as well. But, as we were all grateful to see, with the strength of her positive nature, she adapted. Even more, everyone agreed that the reduction of the UTI events—which could be debilitating—more than made up for the troublesomeness of the medical device.

On a follow-up visit with Dr. Thompson, my mother's Health History sheet was updated. My mother was delighted. Before recording the recent surgery added to her other issues, Dr. Thompson began the baseline paragraph: "Margaret Cottrell is currently ninety-one years old. She is a sprite, but frail, female who is alert, oriented, and cooperative currently. She has no cognitive impairment."

"That's a nice thing to say," my mother said, when Helen read it to her. She rose up from her chair, slightly more wobbly, and grabbed on to her walker. We were going out to lunch today, as we still tried to do once a week.

"I guess I can live with this. I'm learning," she said, looking down at her leg. "But it has, you know, left me with a problem."

Pushing her walker somewhat more slowly than before, she made her way to the coat closet. For all she had been through, however, my mother still looked remarkably fine, thanks to Helen's attentiveness. She was dressed in a crisp pant suit; Helen had helped apply a little lipstick and a touch of rouge to her cheeks. She had recently had her hair done, and Helen fluffed up the back, as it always got flattened to her head from sitting so much in her chair.

The only indication of the collecting bag was a prominent bulge on the outside of her right calf.

"What problem?" I asked.

"These bags…and what they mean."

I looked at my mother, confused.

She sighed and shook her head. Then she stood up straighter, with her spirit of resolve to make the best of things.

"They mean, Marcy, no more dresses."

What I Wish I'd Known

Frailty: What is it?

And How Can You Reduce the Risk of Your Parent— or You—Becoming Frail?

Elizabeth Eckstrom, MD, MPH, MACP

Like many aging seniors, Margaret accumulated more medical issues over time. It was harder for her to rise from a chair; she became more easily fatigued, and began requiring more aids, such as a walker to ambulate, hearing aids, and more help with the activities of daily living. Gradually, she was developing one of the hardest geriatric syndromes to manage: frailty.

Frailty is a condition that is common in older adults, but often goes unrecognized by primary care teams until it is too late to do much about it. Fortunately for Margaret, Dr. Thompson recognized Margaret's early frailty, and offered the best treatment possible—minor surgery to reduce her risk of having more urinary tract infections. And of course, she continued to encourage Margaret to regularly exercise and eat a healthy diet.

What is frailty? How can you recognize it in your parent—or yourself—and what can you do to prevent it? While difficult questions, they are essential to understand if you are helping to care for an older adult— or if you are getting older yourself.

Let's look at them one at a time.

What is frailty?

Frailty, as defined by Dr. Linda Fried—one of the leaders in the field of understanding frailty as a geriatric syndrome, and founder of the Johns Hopkins Center on Aging and Health—has five key components. To be considered frail, you must have three of the five following conditions:

1. Unintentional weight loss
2. Exhaustion
3. Muscle weakness

4. Slowness in walking
5. Low levels of activity

Frailty is a state of diminished reserve—you just don't have as much ability to "bounce back" from small or large setbacks. The most common first symptom of frailty is muscle weakness. Other symptoms follow, with unintentional weight loss and exhaustion usually being the last symptoms to present.

Among people over 65, 7–16 percent who live at home exhibit frailty, a number that increases to 25 percent for those over eighty-five years old.

This presents a problem as people who are frail have increased risk of falls, disability, hospitalizations, and even death.

How do you recognize frailty in your parent or yourself?

Frailty usually begins subtly. It can be so imperceptible, in fact, that even those closest to an older adult may not recognize it right away. Key markers to look for include observing if your parent gradually chooses to walk shorter distances, and with a slower gait. Another early sign is that they may start to have more difficulty getting out of a chair—a result of reduced quadriceps strength. Muscle weakness is a major indicator; even something as non-descript as difficulty opening jars can signal early frailty.

Often, new frailty is a consequence of illness or injury. Persons who were not frail to begin with may spend several days in the hospital with bad pneumonia, a heart attack or an infection, and return home weaker, slower, and with less energy than when they entered the hospital.

Another sign of developing frailty appears to be linked to what experts call reduced "life space,"—in other words, the area that a person moves through during a day and the frequency with which they move. If an older person used to regularly go to church, the hairdresser, occasional shopping trips downtown, out to lunch with friends, and visiting family, that person has a pretty large spatial area. As they get older, however, they may begin limiting travels to just one or two things—signifying a significant reduction in their life space.

Reduction of life space is an indicator of problems ahead. It can lead to decreased physical activity, decreased social engagement, accelerated loss of physical function, and the development of frailty.

Monitoring your loved one for any changes in life space, as well as observing signs of weakness and limited mobility is often the very best way to detect the beginnings of frailty.

What can you do to prevent or reverse frailty in your parent or yourself?

Loss of muscle mass, or sarcopenia, is a major component of muscle weakness and increasing frailty. Is there anything you can do to stop it?

Yes! One of the most potent protectors against sarcopenia is to engage in resistance exercise—which has been shown to improve strength and muscle mass even in people in their nineties!

Practicing yoga, using resistance bands, or lifting light weights at least two to three days per week will help prevent or reduce sarcopenia and help stem the ill effects of frailty.

Recent studies show that following the Mediterranean diet can reduce the risk of developing frailty. It is also important to make sure to consume adequate calories, being especially mindful of eating enough protein. For older persons who have lost their appetite or are quickly satiated when eating, this can be challenging, yet it is essential to keeping frailty at bay. In addition, making sure to get adequate vitamin D—at least 800 IU vitamin D3 daily—is also thought to be important, though the research is not strong in this area.

A critical factor often overlooked by older persons and those who care for them is the negative effects that can be the result of the medications they are taking. It is important, therefore, to always review the drugs your loved one or you are on. A number of medications can cause weakness, fatigue, and other symptoms that are linked to frailty. Prednisone, a powerful anti-inflammatory, and sleeping pills are good examples of drugs that can cause frailty.

Be sure to check the **Beers List, Appendix 1**, for drugs that can cause serious side effects. Also, the British Geriatric Society has a nice web resource called "Fit for Frailty," http://www.bgs.org.uk/frailty -explained/resources/campaigns/fit-for-frailty/frailty-what-is-it for those who are interested in learning more.

In her later years, Margaret had all of the early markers of frailty. As research shows, the syndrome is very hard to reverse once it has taken hold and grown severe. Margaret's hospitalizations, episodes of delirium, and medical history made it truly challenging to prevent frailty. Marcy and the caregivers, though, with the guidance of Dr. Thompson, helped Margaret keep active and engaged in social and cognitive activities to reduce its debilitating progression.

Being on the lookout for early warning signs of frailty, monitoring these markers over time, and using suggested techniques to mitigate frailty's development can assist in reducing the more devastating effects of a frequently overlooked problem, and allow more years of quality of life for your loved one or you.

· *42* ·

How to Pack For the Next Trip

$\mathcal{O}$ne afternoon in early April, when the rhododendrons were beginning to blossom and trilliums dotted the fir forest near her home, my mother sat in her living room talking to her closest neighbor, Geneva Armstrong. Overhearing the two aging seniors from the kitchen, I paused to listen to their interesting conversation:

They were discussing the maxims that Geneva maintained were the secrets to a long, happy life.

Geneva was closing in on one hundred and at this point a legend in the neighborhood. She still lived independently, had been in the same house for nearly seventy years, and loved to travel to the beach, the mountains, and to Hawaii with her son. Geneva said she lived by three simple axioms:

1. Plan ahead.
2. Do your best, then forget about it.
3. Live as though you were going to live forever.

"It takes the stress out of living. Life doesn't have to be perfect and you don't have to do everything all at once," said Geneva, at ninety-eight. "I'm not worried; plus, I've got all the important things all planned, even my one hundredth birthday."

"I think there is something to what Geneva says," said my mother, nearly ninety-two years old, after Geneva walked home.

At her semi-annual check-up, Dr. Thompson continued to be delighted with my mother's condition. "Your mom remains physically very frail, but psychologically she's strong. She obviously wants to be here, and has a good quality of life."

She also brought up to my mother the value of putting things in order, a conversation similar to what she'd had with Geneva. My mother had already formalized many of the planning steps, but the difference was that now my mother talked about them more, and further, wanted to go over them with me. At Dr. Thompson's suggestion, my mother brought up topics like health-care directives, estate planning, naming her personal representative—most of which I didn't like discussing at all. It seemed macabre, somehow, and all about a future I didn't want to face—a life without her in it.

A close friend, though, whose mother was going through the same planning process, had a different outlook. She said her mother had helped her to see that such dialogues weren't gruesome. Rather, they spoke to a plain fact of life. And instead of recoiling from it all, as I tended to do, my friend told me I needed to think about it in a new way.

"It's just another step on this road we are all traveling," she counseled. "Your mother and dad saw many places through the years and had lots of great adventures together. And they didn't go unprepared. Right now what your mom is doing is packing for the next trip."

Helen concurred with my friend, when I brought up the matter with her. She also disclosed that my mother had recently discussed the subject of heaven with her.

"Your mom asked me last week if I believed in life after death. I said yes. She said, 'what do you think happens when you die?' I opened my mouth to say, 'I don't know' but suddenly the words just came over me, I'm not sure where from.

"I said, 'Margaret, I think it's like this: I think it's like when Marcy was little and you and George were going to go somewhere in your plane. You and George were leaving and Marcy didn't want you to go, but at the same time, she wanted you to go, because she knew where you were going was good. It's kind of like that, I think, when we get ready to die. Our families really don't want us to go, because they're going to miss us, but they know it's a journey. You will be getting on an airplane, and when you land there's George, and your Mom and Dad and everyone you've known and loved who's gone before you and I think they're waiting.'

Helen became more thoughtful. "I said, 'Margaret, when the time comes, if you see the plane, if you see the light, go for it! You will wave us good-bye, but they all will be waving you in, on the other side!'"

For a while, there was no more talk of dying, which was a relief, but of living. Emily and Jennifer's lives were accelerating, growing and changing daily, and my mother was swept up in it. She witnessed the joy —and celebration—of Emily getting admitted to medical school, which had been Emily's life long dream. Even better was that Emily had been accepted at Oregon

Health and Sciences University—the same school that her grandfather had attended seventy one years before! In the old administration building on campus, there was a little picture of my father and his graduating class at one end of a long hallway. My mother was happy to think that, at the other end, there would be another little picture, this time of her granddaughter.

Jennifer, too, was rapidly finishing college and still intent on veterinary school. My mother said, "I know she will succeed because she has such a way with animals. I want to live to see it."

Both Emily and Jennifer still loved to spend time with their grandmother when they could. Witnessing the enjoyment crossing back and forth between generations made me reflect on the advantage they had of knowing their grandparents, spending time with them, and listening to their stories.

Stories! The "old ones" offer the young ones chronicles of living. They give us a sense of where we came from and who we are. Like my father's *The Airplane Diaries*, stories remind us how to get along in life and teach us ways to make it through. They offer perspective and, when hard times come, furnish courage and sometimes even direction on how we could respond.

Observing Nana teaching Emily and Jennifer the hula one evening (a little difficult to do with a walker) I saw how a ninety-two year old's stories revealed a depth of knowledge that couldn't be replicated on the Internet. The laughter, the silliness, the memories were relational, with little to do with personal ambition and gain but everything to do with caring and being human.

There had been countless remembrances through the years, many I had already passed on to Emily and Jennifer. I thought I knew them all by heart. But on the sixth anniversary of my father's death, when my mother and I were visiting the cemetery to bring him lilies, she gave me still another.

The day was cool and clear, the flowers my mother held were just budding and smelled sweet. For her and me, the old sadness of visiting his gravesite had lessened over time. Instead, being there conferred a sense of comfort, like we were stopping by for a cozy chat.

"He kept his promise, you know," said my mother, laying the flowers upon his grave. "And he did so faithfully for sixty-one years."

"What promise?" I asked, curiously.

My mother stood erect next to her walker. "The one he made when my mother and father were killed. George was the first to get word after that terrible car crash. I don't know how he kept it from me for as long as he did."

"What do you mean?"

"He got the call at work. I was at home, making him a special dinner. We hadn't been married long and didn't have much then—he was a struggling medical resident," she smiled at the memory, "but we made do. That evening I had set the table with a tablecloth someone had given us for a wedding present, and put out the candlesticks, and made something—I think a pot roast. Your dad worked so hard and such long hours, I wanted him to know how much I appreciated him.

"Well, he came home earlier than I expected, and I was there to greet him. He took in all the effort I had put out, and sat down. He let me serve the dinner, and he ate the entire meal while I talked about all sorts of nonsense, but mostly happy nonsense. He listened, and only after we had finished everything, did he tell me."

"But how did you stand it?" I cried. "You were an only child. You didn't have any children yet. You were suddenly left all alone!"

"It was," she paused, "very hard. I adored my mother and father. People everywhere wrote letters, and many people were also left bereft, including lots of my father's patients. He was their doctor and they loved him. They felt about him like many of your father's patients felt about him. Both were wonderful, caring doctors, like Emily and Jennifer will be. But I wasn't alone, remember. I had George."

Yes, I reflected, she had my dad.

"In a way, it drew us closer. I only had him, and he was there for me. He kept his word."

"What word?" I asked. "What did he pledge to you?"

"It wasn't to me," she replied, "it was to my father. George didn't tell me about it, though, until years later. The night my parents were killed, he wrote a note, saying that he would take care of me and love me and be faithful to me for the rest of my life, to the highest ability that was in him. He placed that note in my father's suit pocket, close to his heart, on the day of my mother and father's funeral."

The scent of flowers was in the air. "And you kept that promise," she said, not to me, but to something I couldn't see. "All your life you kept it. And because of that, I could let my parents go."

Faithful Companion

"The German shepherd dog is back," said Helen, on the other end of the phone. Her voice sounded tired.

"I remember you telling me about it not long after I first started work," she continued. "Well, your mom's starting to see the dog again and talking about it as if it's lying right next to her. I'm wondering if she has a urinary tract infection."

How many years had it been since my mother and I had kidded about her hospital guardian, the German shepherd? Helen wasn't laughing. With the revisiting of this phantom, an old anxiety I hadn't felt for a while began creeping up my spine.

This was not dementia, and it didn't sound like the Charles Bonnet syndrome. My mother knew when she saw things that weren't "real." When she came down with a urinary tract infection, though, it readily impacted her cognition. I had witnessed several episodes when, in five days or less, my mother would go from perfectly well to nearly comatose with overwhelming weakness and confusion.

It was a common occurrence in nursing homes. As I had learned the hard way, numerous people in nursing homes diagnosed with dementia were probably not demented at all—but were suffering from untreated urinary tract infections. Sometimes diminished mental capacity was the primary symptom. I shuddered to think of all the old people wasting away in long-term care facilities that could be enjoying better health if only they had the correct diagnoses.

For two years, Dr. Thompson had successfully kept the severe effects of these infections at bay—treating them quickly and with the appropriate antibiotic therapy.

"If you could get a urine sample, I'll come over and take it to the lab," I told Helen. "I'll call Dr. Thompson right away, and I suspect she'll have us begin antibiotics."

"That will be fine, but I have to say, this seems, well, different," Helen came back. "Your mom's pretty weak. Ever since her ninety-third birthday a couple of weeks ago when your sisters left, she's been asking to sleep more. All morning she keeps repeating to me to make sure the dog has water."

Dr. Thompson didn't appear overly concerned when I finally reached her. She speculated my mother might be fatigued from the company she had staying in town with her for her birthday party. She advised letting her rest, keeping watch, and waiting for the lab results.

When they came back, the bacteria was more serious than Dr. Thompson expected. She started my mother on Cipro, a powerful, broad-spectrum antibiotic. But after a week there was not much improvement. My mother was starting to sleep even more and, even more worrisome to me, when awake, she didn't talk much. She continued seeing the German shepherd dog, who apparently had moved even closer to her chair. It lay so near, in fact, that she could pet it, which she occasionally did.

Dr. Thompson requested a new sample. This one came back negative for the "bad" bacteria, which was good news, but a yeast infection had shown up. She prescribed Diflucan to treat it but also said she wanted to see my mother in her office.

I took her the following day. The doctor carefully listened to her lungs, examined her ears and throat, and took her vital signs.

"I'm a little puzzled," said Dr. Thompson to me, wonderingly. "Her lungs are clear, there's no evidence of aspiration pneumonia, and what we are seeing is not our typical UTI." She faced my mother and took her hand in hers. "How are you feeling, Margaret?"

"Tired," replied my mother, simply.

Dr. Thompson took yet another urine sample, said we should continue with Diflucan, and asked that we watch my mother closely.

After three weeks of antibiotics, my mother's urine was clean of any bacteria. While "cured," her weariness and peculiar behavior had not budged. Worse, she was becoming increasingly confused. She wasn't eating well and took sips of chocolate Ensure—which she previously savored—with reluctance. All she seemed to want to do was sleep and occasionally pet the dog. My alarm growing, I called the doctor again.

Dr. Thompson was thoughtful. "Considering your mother's history, *and* yours, I think we need to be clear on what we are facing," she said. "We need to know the lay of the land. I would like you to take your mother to the ER and get a full workup. I need to see her electrolyte levels and make certain there aren't any other infections setting up shop somewhere."

Dr. Thompson also said she would order a chest x-ray, an enzyme test to see whether my mother may have had a heart attack, a CT scan to check for bleeding on the brain, and yet another urinalysis.

"Have them page me immediately with the results," she concluded firmly.

Patiently and without complaint, my mother undertook the battery of tests. In between workups, as she lay on the hospital gurney, she smiled sweetly at me. "I love you," she whispered.

Panic swept me. I forced it down, convincing myself that with all the tests she was undergoing, we would soon know what was wrong. Then Dr. Thompson would prescribe something, so she would get better. Then we would know what ailed her—it would have a name. Things always seemed more treatable if they had a name. You could look it up and read about it and surf the Internet to find out how other people dealt with it. The web, of course, was not always accurate, more often than not rife with medical misinformation, but at least it meant you were not alone. But my mother's problem did not have a name. To my disappointment and complete surprise, my mother was well. Each test came back negative. All her labs were within proper range. As the emergency room doctor explained it, there was *nothing organically wrong with my mother.*

At the same time, as everyone could see, everything was.

· *44* ·

Crossing the Line

*B*efore my eyes, my mother was fading. But this time my adversary was one I had not encountered before. The rapid demise that I was helplessly observing wasn't the result of a new infection or pneumonia, a hospital-associated disability, uncaring health professionals, or simply being "written off." This was a different scenario altogether, and all the advocating I could pull from my fourteen-year battleground arsenal seemed powerless to stop it.

She slept more and, when awake, began refusing food and water, saying she felt too weak to eat or drink. Concerned that if she didn't get fluids she would not pull through, Dr. Thompson had her admitted to the hospital—the first time in over two years.

Hope pulsed through me when new labs returned, revealing a staph infection of her bladder. This we could deal with. But the method of treatment quickly became barbarous. My mother required IV antibiotics to combat the bacteria, and in her dehydrated state, even expert phlebotomists had trouble finding a proper vein in her arms or legs that didn't rupture when punctured. Soon, my mother was a living pincushion in continual pain from being poked repeatedly with needles, with pockmarks of bruises to prove it erupting all across her arms, hands, and legs. I could not stand witnessing such misery . . . nor could Dr. Thompson, who compassionately prescribed a PICC line once again to spare my mother more suffering.

To my increasing dismay, however, there was minimal improvement after six days of antibiotic therapy in the hospital. Although the bacteria count was greatly reduced, my mother did not rebound. She remained weak, almost continually sleeping. Perplexed, Dr. Thompson said she wished a conference with us to discuss my mother's unexpected condition.

The following day, we arrived for the consultation shortly before one in the afternoon. John had taken time off from work; one of my sisters had driven down from Seattle to meet the doctor; Helen, as always, was there and standing guard. Gathering around my sleeping mother before the doctor arrived, none of us said much. Taking us by surprise, my mother opened her eyes. Seeing all of us assembled, she smiled; her deep brown eyes were amazingly clear.

After days of near muteness, she opened her lips to speak. "Hi, darlings," she said hoarsely.

The sound of the beloved voice brought joy back to my heart. "I'm so happy you're better!" I cried with relief, gently throwing my arms around her. My mother fumbled to take my hand in her frail one. Squeezing it lightly, she gazed at each one of us in turn. With her macular degeneration, I could not be sure what she saw, but the love in her eyes was unmistakable. What she said next, though, almost pummeled me to the floor.

"I'm ready to go," she whispered.

I could not have heard correctly.

My sister blanched, Helen looked stern, and John stared at me. At that moment, Dr. Thompson entered the room. She knew something had just happened from observing our faces and quickly strode over to my mother. She touched her. My mother, still smiling radiantly, glanced at Dr. Thompson and then repeated the same disastrous phrase to her.

Dr. Thompson waited momentarily before speaking. She regarded my mother closely, then lowered her face close to hers. Very gently, and so softly it seemed to be for my mother's ears alone, she asked, tenderly, "Are you saying, Margaret, you feel ready to go to heaven?"

"Yes," replied my mother, closing her eyes.

The room was suddenly blurry. I knew I had just dreamed this whole thing. I needed to wake up and start over again. "Let's step into the hall," Dr. Thompson was motioning.

I took in my mother's peace-filled face with a sense of horror. Helen lightly nudged me to follow the procession out the door.

"This was not the conference I was expecting," admitted Dr. Thompson as we stood, dumbstruck, around her. "I am as astonished as you are. Even though we have been giving her continual antibiotics for nearly a month to treat very mild infections, the treatment is not effective."

"But why aren't the antibiotics working?" I asked, feeling helpless. "Does she need a different drug, like the last time?"

"They aren't working because there is nothing inherently wrong with your mother."

"But doesn't she have an infection?"

"The infection has cleared."

"Then why is she acting like this? Sleeping so much? Saying things like . . . well, like she just said?" I persisted. "She must have an infection to be so confused!"

"Did she look confused to you?" asked Dr. Thompson, gently.

My throat constricted with the awful truth. No. She appeared completely lucid. I did not answer.

Dr. Thompson gave us several minutes to digest all that had just transpired before offering her opinion. At last she spoke to everyone, but her eyes were upon me. "Although it is very difficult to accept, judging from what your mother has just conveyed, at the same time witnessing her diminishing capacity, I believe we have reached a new point. I call it '*the line in the sand.*'"

None of us could hold back tears now. John put his arm around my shoulder.

"After you cross it," said Dr. Thompson, "your life becomes different."

Her words stood still in the air. The line in the sand? So what did *that* mean? Was she intimating my mother stepped over it? Had *I*? Instinctively, I pulled my feet back under me. I wanted nothing to do with lines.

Dr. Thompson was saying something more; my sister was nodding and asking questions. I heard the term "hospice," and a sickening feeling whirled around me. Hospice? It was a word I didn't want used in the same breath as my mother's name. "Doesn't hospice mean you're *dying*?" I interrupted stupidly.

Dr. Thompson faced me; the compassion on her face was more profound than I'd seen there before. "Hospice is palliative care," she explained. "It means we want your mother to be made comfortable. But even now, it doesn't mean we've given up all hope. Some people mistakenly think that hospice is a one-way destination and that by invoking it, there is no way out except to die. That isn't true. Sometimes patients improve, and then they are removed from hospice care. The trip can go both ways."

I must not have looked convinced. The doctor poised her next words carefully. "Don't let the words 'hospice' or 'palliative care' frighten you. Truly, they are gifts to a very ill patient and to their families. Hospice is there to help you and also to help me—as your mother's physician—to give the kindest, most sympathetic care with the least possible suffering at a critical point in my patient's life."

The words still alarmed me, but what Dr. Thompson did next made me realize she had my mother's best interests front and center in her consideration. She was not Dr. Hip—evicting my mother from the hospital and sending her to a nursing home to die. Dr. Thompson was, rather, *freeing her to go home.*

"Your mother doesn't need to be in the hospital to continue receiving treatment. She has her PICC line, and there are visiting nurses. Although her bacterial count is subclinical, I still intend to manage it."

My sister appeared perplexed, but I knew why Dr. Thompson was continuing her drug therapy. It was not only for my mother, but for *me*. It was a testimony that we weren't giving up. Somehow it made all that she was relating more bearable.

"Your mother has always said she loved being home," continued Dr. Thompson. "Knowing her wishes, I would prefer having her be in her own home, where she can have IV fluids and antibiotics for a time. This will give her one last fighting chance."

"*Is* there any chance?" my sister mumbled.

Dr. Thompson's solemn gray eyes were thoughtful. "I believe we have crossed over the line. From now on, it's not up to us. Margaret's own body is leading the way."

The following day, at noon, we went home. Dr. Thompson was right about one thing: There was a sense of peace for all of us having my mother in her own bed, in the room she loved to be in, where the autumn sun could shine its golden October luminescence on her thinning face.

Visiting nurses were arranged and prepared my mother's vancomycin and fluids. Later in the week, two hospice workers arrived to tell us about their services. The assistance they offered was plentiful. Now that my mother was enrolled, all her medical care, they said, was free. They could manage her pain and drugs, if necessary, and assist as caregivers. Helen, however, boldly announced that she intended to stay with my mother, night and day, around the clock during this time, acting as my mother's personal nurse. I concurred, explaining we desired to be the ones caring for her. The hospice team respectfully assured us that our desires were to be preferred but wished us to know that should we want them, they would be here . . . as things unfolded.

After seven days of infusions, Dr. Thompson asked for another urine and blood sample. Although my mother was dosed with powerful, broad-spectrum drugs and was fully hydrated, she had become only weaker and was now sleeping even more. As odd as it seemed, I found myself desperately hoping the newest labs would show that my mother had a raging infection causing her worrisome symptoms. But when Dr. Thompson called with the latest results, she explained there was absolutely no trace of bacteria in her urine or anywhere in her body or bloodstream.

Then she asked to talk to me for a moment. With an impending sense of doom, I sat down on the couch.

"You have done a great job advocating, you know," she began, "and have kept it up for many years. You've helped give both of your parents a good quality of life."

I didn't want to hear any more. Yet I couldn't help remembering the promise I had made to her, back when things were going well, that I would be able to let my mother go when Dr. Thompson truly felt it was her time. She had saved my mother's life several times, and I believed that she would again if there were any hope. From her tone, though, I gathered that the news was not good.

The sand was shifting beneath my feet. The line was getting closer. Dr. Thompson was pulling me nearer to it.

"In my heart of hearts," said Dr. Thompson, "I feel—it's time."

She waited a few seconds before speaking again. A side of me wanted to shout, "I renege on my promise!" But, deeper than that, on an honest yet terrible level, I knew her words were true.

"Your mother has been on antibiotics for over a month, and she has been infection free for nearly that long. But, as you observe, she continues to decline. As your mother's physician, I do not believe it is right to just 'half-treat' her, in her condition where she can't get any better but continues to get worse."

Her words strangely echoed what Dr. Hobbs had offered me seven years before, when my father lay dying from Alzheimer's. He had said that to rush my father to an emergency room for a "pull-out-all-stops" workup would, in his opinion, be cruel, especially to one so deeply confused.

"Your father has pneumonia," he had counseled, "and there is a slight chance that we might be able to pull him through this time, although I sorely doubt it at this late stage of Alzheimer's disease. But even if we did, another infection would be right on its heels. The short-term 'cure' would be terrifying for him. Let him go in peace. *It is time.*"

Dr. Thompson was saying the same thing, but the circumstances were different. This time, we weren't facing the enemy of an overwhelming viral or bacterial infection. The fact was, my mother's body was at last giving out.

"To continue to treat your mother, I would have to send her to the emergency room again and do more cultures, blood work, and perhaps give her more antibiotics, almost as a placebo," she continued. "But by doing that, I fear that your mother's mental status would continue to worsen to a very scary place for her."

I had vivid recollections of that appalling place. I remembered too well when she had been fraught with delirium. The last thing I wanted was for my mother to pass away—in fear.

"I want to explain something to you," said Dr. Thompson. "Two things are working in tandem here. One is a physiological process. The other is psychological. Previously when your mother was very sick, she had the *psy-*

chological oomph to triumph over the *physiological disease*. In other words, her will to live was stronger than what was trying to take over her body. She was able to tip the scales by the strength of her mind. But there comes a time in everyone's life when that no longer is possible. Now, even if your mother had the psychological will, her own body physiologically can't allow it."

What she said made sense, even though hearing it stabbed me with anguish. So much of life, I knew, was a mind/body connection.

"Up until now, I have felt it right to treat your mother, for I knew that was what she wanted and also that she still had a good quality of life. But though there are a few last half-hearted measures I could still do, I don't feel anymore that it would be right. Your mother has spoken her wishes. I would hope, as her physician, to honor that."

Dr. Thompson paused, as if to let me have time to take in the import of what she was conveying. I knew my mother didn't want feeding tubes or breathing apparatuses or being plied with more and more medicines that couldn't do any good. Yet it seemed wrong, somehow. Wrong to quit fighting. That would be giving up and giving in, wouldn't it? Advocating for my loved ones was what I did and had practiced for the past fourteen years! How could I stop now? How could I really let go?

Dr. Thompson understood my grief. Then she addressed it with the one answer I needed.

"At these times we may think we are making a difference in the outcome, but we are not. We imagine we are making decisions and that we have control. But there comes a time in everyone's life when the decisions we believe we are making really aren't our decisions at all. After we have crossed this line, it is not up to you, nor me, any longer. From here on, it is up to your mother. *She* is leading the way."

On a level deeper than the wishes of my own heart, I knew Dr. Thompson was right. My mother was on the front lines now. She was going forward in grace. I could barely form the words. "How long?"

"Once the IVs and fluids are removed, anywhere from three to fourteen days."

Through her wisdom and sympathy, Dr. Thompson was extending her hand, reaching out for me to take her grasp. With nowhere left to go, I leaned toward her as she lifted me up and helped me to cross the line in the sand. Once on the other side, I was met with searing pain, mingled strangely with a confounding sense of relief. My years of battle, I knew, at last were over. Dr. Thompson was my mother's physician. She was our ally. She was the ally for all old people, giving them respect and dignity until the end.

For that good and noble cause, I knew she would continue the fight, even as I let it go.

What Is Palliative Care, and How Can It Help My Parents and Me?

Elizabeth Eckstrom, MD, MPH, MACP

Palliative care is the most important thing I do as a geriatrician. The word "palliative" comes from the Latin word *palliare*, which means "to cloak." Providing palliative care is literally cloaking a patient and the patient's family with comfort, symptom relief, and love. It doesn't matter whether an older person is very ill and dying or perfectly healthy. Helping that person feel *good* is the overarching goal. Palliative care means stopping medications that cause side effects, starting medications that relieve symptoms like pain, and utilizing diverse therapies such as art therapy, relaxation techniques, and massage to improve physical and mental health.

Yet sometimes palliative care is misconstrued and erroneously thought of as "doing nothing." This may seem particularly so when it concerns your parent. In these cases, it is natural to want your doctor to "do everything." Marcy felt this way for a long time. She advocated for her mother to have more tests, receive more antibiotics, see more specialists. And this was a very understandable reaction for her—especially because both her dad and her mom had been treated with disrespect in the past. Often we equate the acts of conducting more tests, prescribing more medications, doing more surgeries, administering more chemotherapy, and so on with the feeling that our parent is being respected. Sometimes, though, our good intentions can backfire. Sometimes our intensive interventions can cause more pain and distress, such as when Margaret was in the hospital with both arms and legs bruised from having so many people attempting to place an IV in her.

In reality, palliative care is truly "doing everything" for the patient. With palliative care, doctors use their entire team to ensure a person is comfortable and in his or her preferred environment. For example, Marcy's mother had been in emergency rooms and hospitals frequently, but once she started receiving palliative care by Dr. Thompson, she made far fewer trips to the hospital and was able to spend much more time at home. She was able to enjoy her family, take trips with Helen, and go shopping and to lunch. Because Dr. Thompson was skillfully able to remove many offending medications, focus on Margaret's goals, and help educate Marcy and her family, Margaret was able to have a much higher quality of life during her last two years than she might have had otherwise.

Are you surprised I refer to the care Dr. Thompson provided Margaret as *palliative care*? You shouldn't be, for that is exactly what it was, right from the start. It was minimizing risky drugs, focusing on the whole person, and developing a trusting relationship with Margaret and Marcy so that they could *work together* to enhance Margaret's quality of life. Every older person, sick or well, near to death or years away, deserves that humane approach!

Providing palliative care does *not* mean a doctor won't try to cure something when possible. When Margaret had a urinary tract infection, Dr. Thompson prescribed antibiotics to cure it. With palliative care, if you break your hip, you will still have the operation to give you a new hip—because without the operation, you will remain in pain. With palliative care, you may still get cancer treatment, such as radiation, to decrease the pain of the tumor. With palliative care, you don't have to give up hope of living longer. Rather, your focus undergoes a shift—your goal is having the best possible day *today*.

What makes palliative care different? It is that with palliative care, no one will push you to do a treatment that will most likely be futile. For example, if you have cancer and chemotherapy has not been helping but instead is making you miserable, your doctor will not pressure you to attempt yet another type of chemotherapy. If your heart isn't doing well, your doctor will abstain from encouraging you to undergo one more surgery just in case there is "something else" that might help . . . when you both know there isn't. Interestingly, research shows that this palliative approach does not necessarily make you die sooner! Conversely, receiving good palliative care helps to relieve pain and distress from symptoms—*which allows our bodies to focus on healing and longevity.*

A study published in the *New England Journal of Medicine* in 2010 showed that people with lung cancer who got early palliative care had better quality of life and lived nearly three months longer than those who received only cancer treatment without the palliative care. Other research confirmed that those who continued to push for the most aggressive treatment in the last week of life actually had the *poorest* quality of life . . . and who wants that for your parent?

So where does "hospice" fit in the spectrum of palliative care? Hospice is for anyone who is reaching the end of life, whether that person be young or old. Hospice is the ultimate in palliative care—nurses, music therapists, social workers, and many other team members can come directly to your home twenty-four hours a day to ensure you are comfortable. Hospice teams "do everything" to ensure comfort and quality of life, peace for the patient and family, and communication with the healthcare team. Only people whose doctor has deemed them to be in the last six months of their life are eligible for hospice, so the primary doctor is responsible for providing palliative care up until that time. Lots of patients do much better after they start hospice and receive its abundance of services. Some even "graduate" from hospice because they improve so much that they will most likely live far longer than six months.

Luckily, neither of Marcy's parents had a devastating cancer or end-stage lung or heart problems. Marcy's father got palliative care from Dr. Hobbs and died peacefully. Marcy's mother benefited greatly from the palliative care provided by Dr. Thompson. The geriatrician knew when Margaret was approaching life's end so that she could call in hospice to help with all the little details of keeping her comfortable. And because she had developed a relationship of trust with Margaret and Marcy, Dr. Thompson provided the kindness and understanding Marcy desperately needed toward the end of her mother's life.

Dr. Atul Gawande, a renowned physician, captured the true meaning of palliative care in his now famous *New Yorker* story. His words speak what most geriatricians and their teams believe:

> Our responsibility, in medicine, is to deal with human beings as they are. People die only once. They have no experience to draw upon. They need doctors and nurses who are willing to have the hard discussions and say what they have seen, who will help people prepare for what is to come.

· 45 ·

A Good Ending

$\mathcal{T}$he day after Dr. Thompson's call, two visiting nurses arrived to remove my mother's PICC line and unhook her from all IV tethers. With visible relief to be freed from machines and tubes, my mother peacefully accepted the discontinuance of her vancomycin and IV fluids. While nearly everyone who cared for her and loved her traveled with her in agreement, my own passage was not as straightforward.

In short, I jumped back and forth over the line hundreds of times. Sometimes only seconds apart, I alternated from consciously letting her go to grabbing her back again, wanting to save her.

Through it all, she mostly slept. But the moments she was awake, she was clear eyed and lucid. Those times were sacred. She was in no pain. She had no bedsores. Helen carefully tended to her every bodily need, turning her gently, keeping her spotlessly clean, brushing her hair, putting on a little lipstick, dressing her in her favorite nightgowns.

I took time off from everything just to be there all day long in case her eyes opened . . . in case she might utter some final words or give me one of her heartrending smiles. Each smile I locked in my heart, wanting to keep it there always, to be able to retrieve it to my memory when she was no longer here.

Helen purchased a large candle that we lit and kept burning night and day on the table near her bed. We played soft music continually on the CD player. Day after day, the sun streamed into her room, illuminating a strange radiance to her face I had never before witnessed. She was happy she was home—the home she had built with my father and where she had raised her family. Now she was dying in the place she loved best in all the world.

My older sisters, Ann and Karen, came to stay for two weeks to be with her. Emily stopped by every day after medical school. Jennifer drove up from college on the weekends and, during the second week, was excused from classes to spend the days with her grandmother. Other family members and close friends dropped by just to sit with her. Sometimes my mother was awake; most of the time she was not, but everyone felt that even in her diminishing repose, she knew they were there. One especially close friend of my mother's said to me, "Everyone who knew your mother loved her. Of how many people can that be said!"

My favorite moments, though, were when I was by myself at her bedside. These were the private hours I would write in my journal, stare at her face, and sometimes speak what was really in my heart. Alone with her, while she slept, I could whisper my conflicted feelings. Sometimes I would cry. Sometimes I would laugh and reminisce over stories of fun times we shared. At the poignant times when she appeared the most fragile and vulnerable, I would carefully lie next to her and wrap my arms around her. Emily or Jennifer spent hours with her, too, and often sat on my lap next to their beloved grandmother's bed, and we would cry together. But one thing was clear—Dr. Thompson was right. Through it all, my mother *was* leading the way.

While there was great sadness, there were special, happy times, too. One weekend afternoon when my mother was awake and actually perky, Emily washed her hair. She and Helen dried, set, and combed it. They put some makeup and lipstick on my mother, making her beautiful. At the same time, no one could miss observing her high cheekbones were becoming more pronounced and her skin more transparent. When they visited, both Emily and Jennifer also played music for her on the old Steinway piano that was just outside my mother's room. She loved hearing them play, especially the familiar old hymns that indeed lent a sweetness around the house, giving us all a degree of solace.

Days passed slowly, one upon the other, and someone was always at my mother's side. It didn't matter whether she were sleeping or not—everyone talked with her anyway. My sisters would converse about their work and travels and what was going on in their homes. I often read out of my father's book, *The Airplane Diaries*, which, if she were awake, would always make my mother smile. Each evening Emily would tell Nana what she had learned in medical school that day. When her grandmother asked, Emily loved to show her the stethoscope that Nana had bought for her and had engraved with her name. Jennifer visited often and talked about the goings-on of her senior year in college and her happiness in learning she'd been accepted to her favorite school: Washington State University School of Veterinary Medicine. On the heels of all these visits, though, were always breakdown times for Jennifer and Emily—the knowledge that their beloved Nana would most likely not be there to see either one graduate.

On the few occasions my mother actually had an appetite, I loved making her an egg and feeding it to her. But she really was not hungry and refused to eat most of the time, except for when Inez and Alonzo visited. When they came, they always brought her a chocolate shake and an almond croissant from St. Honore. If my mother was awake, she would attempt to take a sip and a tiny bite or two—for them.

"See; she still likes almond croissants! They are good for her!" Alonzo would clap his hands and exclaim through his tears.

While there was support in numbers and a growing acceptance among many that inevitable change was near, the ground beneath my own feet continued to sway. While others sat back to wait, I still yearned to move! To climb that mountain, face my enemy, and defy the specter of death! John understood. And, more than any other, it was to John I turned. As he had always been, he remained the firm rock that could steady the shifting earth. Every night after work, he would sit by my mother and next to me, telling her stories that could make her laugh or, if she were asleep, could make *me* laugh. Just having him near gave all of us courage.

But he did something more. One quiet evening when he and I were alone with her, John made my mother a pledge, not unlike one she had heard before. He promised her he would always be there to take care of me, giving her his word that he would love and cherish me for the rest of our lives.

It was the only time in those final eleven days I saw tears on my mother's face. She held his hand, my hand. John was crying too.

My husband, at that moment, had never looked more beautiful to me.

This book, as it began, ends as a love story. At the beginning of the second week, the days became outlined with an increasingly ethereal quality at the same time my mother's breathing started to thin. One side of me wanted to embrace that otherworldliness, but another continued to resist it. I knew what it meant—she was going somewhere I could not follow. Hospice continued to check her status and monitor her drugs and any pain relief; their grief counselors helped to sustain me when the fine line between life and death seemed unbearable. Dr. Thompson called routinely, making sure my mother was comfortable. Jennifer came home from school. Emily, when not at medical school, joined Jennifer to sit with her grandmother.

In the evenings, everyone gathered around in a passel of chairs arranged around my mother's bed and had dinner in her room while she slept. No one ever wanted to leave, and often we would stay there until nearly twelve, when at last the girls, John, and I would go home and my sisters would go to their rooms to sleep. Helen kept up her twenty-four-hour-a-day vigil, even to the point of sleeping with one ear propped next to the monitor she kept by her own bed, lest my mother need anything in the night.

The hours between one and six in the morning were, for me, the hardest of all. Each time I left I worried that I would get that dreaded call at 3:00 a.m., but the next morning when I arrived, my mother was always there, resting peacefully.

At midnight on the eve of the twelfth day, we prepared, as we always did, to go home. John put on his coat and handed mine to me. I placed one arm through the sleeve, but something made me pause.

"I think I don't want to go," I said, taking off my coat and laying it back on the chair. "Why don't you take the girls home? I'll sleep here."

John looked surprised, then reluctant. "Do you want me to stay?"

"No; I'm fine. You need to go home and feed the animals. It's already late. I'll come home first thing in the morning."

Helen had already gone to bed; my sisters were preparing to. Emily and Jennifer, however, picking up on my change in mood, voiced that they would like to stay with me.

"No, go home and stay with Dad. I appreciate it, but you'll sleep better there."

"Where will *you* sleep?" John queried.

"I'll make do—with the couch and a blanket."

My mother was resting on her back, dressed in her prettiest pink satin nightgown. Though her respirations were somewhat labored, she appeared tranquil. "All right," he agreed at last, with hesitation. "I'll see you in the morning." Then he bent down and gave my mother a kiss on her forehead.

"Nana still looks so beautiful!" said Emily, kissing her too. She could not hold back her tears.

Jennifer leaned over and hugged her. "I love you so much, Nana."

In the pale light from the burning candle and night light by her bed, my mother's face indeed reflected a loveliness that did not seem to diminish, but to grow. The serenity and calmness on her face only augmented the steady ache in my anxious heart.

"Well, I hope *you* get some sleep," said John, frowning. "You look totally worn out, Mar."

"Don't worry; I'll sleep. And I'm not the only one who looks tired," I smiled at him. But after they left, I could not rest right away. For whatever reason, my eyes would not release from my mother. Karen came back into the room, wondering why I was still there. She sat down in the chair next to me and picked up my mother's soft hand. Both of us noted that her breathing sounded worse, with longer pauses in between. Ann, passing by the room and spying us, entered and sat down too.

The night dragged, the candlelight flickered, and all of us had difficulty staying awake. "You go to bed," I said to my sisters. "I'm about to head for the couch. It's just that I don't want to leave her." Suddenly, I was struck with an idea. "Well, I don't *have* to leave her. I'll just bring some cushions from the couch in here."

"You're going to sleep by her bed?" asked Karen.

I yawned. "Uh-huh."

"I like that idea," said Karen. "I don't want to leave her either. There are plenty of pads and blankets. I'll bring some in for me too."

"If you both are, then I will too!" exclaimed Ann, surprisingly awake. "We can have a slumber party!"

The image, probably exaggerated by our altered mental states at two in the morning, was appealing. A slumber party with my sisters and mother was something that actually sounded like fun.

"We can bring in *all* the cushions and sleep on the floor by Mother's bed!" Ann was saying. "We'll move Mother directly into the center of the room, so we can sleep on every side of her."

Like twelve-year-olds, we dashed for the living room and then to the linen closet, pulling cushions off the couches and grabbing out bedding, unmindful whether extra sheets and pillowcases fell on the floor as we snatched them from the shelves. Soon the floor of my mother's room was a mess of pads, bolsters, throw rugs, pillows, and coverlets. We were all laughing now.

"Mom," explained Ann, pulling up the hospital bed rails, "we have to disturb you just for a moment to wheel you to the middle of the room." Gripping the handles, she tried pushing the bed. When it didn't budge, she heaved it some more.

"What's wrong? Why won't this thing *move?*"

"Because you have the brakes on!" cried Karen, coming to the other side of the bed and releasing the guard. "Quit forcing it! Stop jostling Mother!" Ann, however, was nearly doubled over in hysterics. "Haven't you learned anything about hospital beds after these weeks?" said Karen, shaking her head.

But Karen could not hold back her laughter either. "Okay, let's do this together," she said, clutching a rail. We each took hold, giggling even harder, and shoved the cot with our mother in it over strewn blankets and some pillows until it was situated properly in the room's center. My mother, still fast asleep, was breathing softly.

"There!" I said, still unable to stop laughing. Carefully, we pulled up my mother's covers again and then arranged all the cushions in a circle around her bed. "We're going to have a real slumber party, Mom, and *you* are the guest of honor!"

In some way none of us could explain, my mother seemed to be enjoying herself, taking everything in stride. For the first time in weeks, the atmosphere of the room felt lighthearted and gay.

"Look, I think Mother is smiling!" said Karen, though she really couldn't see too much in the candlelight.

"Let's go change, and then we can come back in for the party. I've got some old PJs in my bedroom closet," I said, hurriedly pushing my cushion almost directly under my mother's bed; I wanted to make sure I was the closest. "We'll all be right back, Mom. Don't go away!"

"How *could* Mother go anywhere—with so much stuff piled up all around her bed?" said Ann.

Following after me, she and Karen found their nightgowns and went to my mother's bathroom to change. For the next five minutes, the small, pink-tiled room was a gaggle of three sisters talking and laughing, dressing in pajamas and brushing their teeth. It was like the old happy times in the house—when everyone was home and prattling and just enjoying each other.

"Mar," Karen called from the other room, having left us only a moment before. I tuned my ears to listen at the same time Ann was making faces at me as I struggled to put my arms in an ugly old nightgown I hadn't worn in years. I had it on backward.

"What?" I yelled to the other room, trying unsuccessfully to yank it off over my head. "I'm *coming*! Has the party started?"

"Mar . . . Ann," Karen called again, calm and low. "Mother stopped breathing."

Parents give us many things. They give us life and love. They show us how to laugh and when to cry and, for many of us, how to follow our dreams, positively embrace life, and trust in a compassionate God. Mine taught me what it meant to remain faithful to others throughout a lifetime—in times of health and sickness, happiness and sorrow, through their courage and grace, without judging.

Unquestioningly, my parents gave me far more than I could ever have repaid and without thought of return. But in the weeks and months after their passing, I came to realize there was one thing I felt grateful to have provided them.

Looking back, I saw how I had been blessed with the privilege to help give the parents I so loved *a good ending*.

Appendix 1

The Drugs Seniors Should Not Be On but Are Too Often Prescribed, as Determined by the American Geriatric Society "Beers List"

ELIZABETH ECKSTROM, MD, MPH, MACP

with David S. H. Lee, PharmD, PhD (Oregon State University/ Oregon Health Sciences University) and Allison Gille

*T*he following list of drugs (generic names in bold; brand names in italics) should not be used in older adults. A key to their adverse effects is included with each drug. If these medications are prescribed, patients should consult with their doctor to determine whether the medication is appropriate or whether it should be switched to a different medication. As with all drugs, patients should question their doctors each time a new drug is prescribed:

What is the drug for?
What side effects could it cause?
How will we know it is working?
When will the drug be stopped?
How will we monitor for side effects?
What other medications could this medication interact with, and how can I assure that it doesn't happen to me?

A
Acetylcholinesterase inhibitors: 11, 17
Actos: 37
Advil: 35, 37, 43, 56
Aldactone: 4, 15
Aldomet: 8, 11, 48
Aldoril: 8, 11, 48
Aleve: 35, 37, 43, 56
Alprazolam: 19, 39, 46, 54, 55
Ambien: 22, 39, 46, 55
Amiodarone: 3, 4, 17, 32, 49

Amitriptyline: 2, 3, 8, 39, 42, 45, 46, 54, 55, 59, 64
Amobarbital: 18, 19, 39, 46, 50, 51, 54, 55
Amphetamine: 40
Amrix: 2, 39, 42, 45, 54
Amytal: 18, 19, 39, 46, 50, 51, 55
Anafranil: 2, 3, 8, 39, 42, 45, 46, 55, 59, 64
Anaspaz: 2, 5, 6, 39, 42, 45, 46, 54, 55
Androderm: 23, 24

Feldene: 35, 37, 43, 56
Fenoprofen: 35, 37, 43, 56
Fesoterodine: 2, 39, 42, 54, 55
Fexmid: 2, 39, 42, 45, 54
Fioricet: 18, 19, 39, 40, 46, 50, 51, 54, 55
Fiorinal: 18, 19, 39, 40, 46, 50, 51, 54, 55
First-generation antihistamines: 1, 2, 3, 4, 39, 42, 45, 46, 54, 55
Flecainide: 3, 11, 49
Flexeril: 2, 39, 42, 45, 54
Flexon: 2, 39, 42, 45, 54, 55
Flurazepam: 19, 39, 46, 54, 55
Fortesta: 23, 24
Furadantin: 3, 10, 61

G
Glyburide: 3, 29, 64
Glynase: 3, 29, 64
Growth hormone: 26
Guanabenz: 8, 11, 48
Guanfacine: 8, 11, 48

H
Halcion: 19, 39, 46, 54, 55
H2-receptor antagonists: 39
Hydramine: 1, 2, 3, 4, 39, 42, 45, 46, 54, 55
Hydroxyzine: 2, 3, 4, 39, 42, 45, 54, 55
HyoMax: 2, 5, 6, 39, 42, 45, 46, 54, 55
Hyoscine: 2, 5, 6, 39, 42, 45, 54, 55
Hyoscyamine: 2, 5, 6, 39, 42, 45, 46, 54, 55
Hytrin: 3, 8, 44, 48

I
Ibuprofen: 35, 37, 43, 56
Ibutilide: 3, 11, 49
Imipramine: 2, 3, 8, 39, 42, 45, 46, 54, 55, 59, 64
Indocin: 35, 37, 43, 56
Indomethacin: 35, 37, 43, 56
Insulin, sliding scale: 27
Intermezzo: 22, 39, 46, 55
Intuniv, extended release: 8, 11, 48

Isofed: 40
Isoptin: 37, 42
Isoxsuprine: 52

K
Kapvay: 8, 11, 48
Ketoprofen: 35, 37, 43, 56
Ketorolac: 35, 37, 43, 56
Klonopin: 19, 39, 46, 54, 55

L
Lanoxin: 4, 11, 13, 39, 49
Lentizol: 2, 3, 8, 39, 42, 45, 46, 54, 55, 59, 64
Levbid: 2, 5, 6, 39, 42, 45, 46, 54, 55
Levo-duboisine: 2, 5, 6, 39, 42, 45, 54, 55
Levsin: 2, 5, 6, 39, 42, 45, 46, 54, 55
Librax: 2, 5, 6, 19, 39, 42, 45, 46, 54, 55
Librium: 19, 39, 46, 54, 55
Limbitrol: 2, 3, 8, 19, 39, 42, 45, 46, 54, 55, 59, 64
Lodine: 35, 37, 43, 56
Lodrane: 2, 3, 4, 39, 40, 42, 45, 46, 54, 55
Lorazepam: 19, 39, 46, 54, 55
Lorzone: 2, 54
Ludiomil: 2, 3, 38, 39, 42, 45, 54, 55
Lunesta: 22, 39, 46, 55

M
Macrobid: 3, 10, 61
Macrodantin: 3, 10, 61
Maprotiline: 2, 3, 38, 39, 42, 45, 54, 55
Martifur-MR: 3, 10, 61
Masmoran: 2, 3, 4, 39, 42, 45, 54, 55
Mebaral: 18, 19, 39, 46, 50, 51, 54, 55
Meclastin: 2, 3, 4, 39, 42, 45, 46, 54, 55
Meclofenamate: 35, 37, 43, 56
Mefenamic acid: 35, 37, 43, 56
Megace: 28
Megestrol: 28
Mellaril: 2, 8, 11, 16, 17, 38, 39, 41, 42, 45, 46, 54, 55, 59, 64
Meloxicam: 35, 37, 43, 56

Key to Risks

Reference Number	
1	Use in special situations—such as treating severe allergic reactions—may be appropriate
2	Can cause confusion, drowsiness, blurred vision, difficulty urinating, dry mouth, and constipation
3	Safer medications available that may provide better results or cause fewer side effects, or both
4	Drug's clearance through the system is reduced with patient's advancing age
5	Not clear whether these drugs are effective
6	Avoid except in short-term palliative care to decrease oral secretions
7	Antithrombotics—drugs to prevent or dissolve blood clots
8	Can make blood pressure drop when standing up ("orthostatic hypotension"); this can cause dizziness and lead to dangerous falls
9	More effective agents available for treatment of Parkinson's disease
10	May cause side effects that affect the lungs
11	May cause a slow heartbeat and dizziness
12	May increase risk of heart failure in older adults
13	In heart failure, higher doses seem to have no additional benefit and may increase risk of toxicity, especially in patients with kidney problems
14	May lower blood pressure
15	In people with heart failure, higher doses may boost risk of high potassium
16	Increased risk of stroke; may increase risk of death in persons with dementia
17	May increase risk of dangerous changes in heartbeat
18	Over time, less effective in helping older adults sleep
19	Do not use for treating insomnia, agitation, or delirium May increase risk of mental decline, delirium, falls, fractures, and car accidents in older adults May be appropriate, however, in some cases for treating seizures and end-of-life care
20	Not effective long term; high risk of overdose
21	Makes older adults sleepy

Reference Number	
22	May not significantly improve sleep Can cause confusion, falls, delirium, and bone fractures Avoid long-term use (over ninety days)
23	May cause or worsen heart problems
24	Should not be prescribed for men with prostate cancer
25	May increase risk of breast cancer and cancer of the lining of the uterus Do not appear to help protect women from heart disease or loss of thinking ability in later life Topical vaginal cream is acceptable at low doses
26	Can cause joint pain, swelling, enlargement of breast tissue in men, and carpal tunnel syndrome
	May also increase the chance of getting diabetes
27	Not an effective way to dose insulin Can increase chance of low blood sugar
28	Prescribed to increase appetite but not very effective May increase chance of blood clots and possibly death
29	Can cause dangerous low blood sugar in older adults
30	May cause shakiness, sleepiness, and uncontrollable abnormal body movements, especially in frail older adults
31	Not a very effective pain reliever and may cause seizures
32	May contribute to thyroid, lung, and heart problems
33	Potential to cause aspiration pneumonia
34	Not very effective for treating vomiting
35	Can increase risk of GI bleeding/peptic ulcer disease in high-risk groups, including those over seventy-five
36	Can cause confusion and hallucinations
37	Potential to promote fluid retention and/or exacerbate heart failure in seniors with heart failure
38	Lowers seizure threshold in seniors with epilepsy or suffering chronic seizures
39	May induce or worsen delirium in older adults at risk of delirium
40	Avoid in persons suffering from insomnia; drug acts as a stimulant
41	Potential to worsen Parkinsonian symptoms in people with Parkinson's disease

Reference Number	
42	Can worsen constipation in seniors suffering from chronic constipation
43	May increase risk of acute kidney injury in persons with chronic kidney disease stages IV and V
44	Avoid in women who suffer from incontinence May aggravate incontinence
45	Avoid in men with an enlarged prostate May decrease urinary flow and cause urinary retention
46	May worsen episodes of falling in individuals with a history of falling
47	Antispasmodics—drugs prescribed to relieve cramps or spasms
48	Not recommended for treatment of high blood pressure
49	Should not be first choice for treating atrial fibrillation
50	Can cause physical dependence
51	Greater risk of overdose at lower doses
52	Not effective
53	May not be appropriate for patients with a history of heart problems
54	Increased risk of fractures
55	May produce lack of coordination of muscle movements in seniors with history of falling
56	May exacerbate existing ulcers or cause new ones in people with history of gastric or duodenal ulcers
57	*Use with caution* in adults eighty years and older Lack of evidence of benefit versus risk
58	*Use with caution* in adults seventy-five years and older Greater risk of bleeding in older adults
59	*Use with caution in older adults* May worsen or cause excess water accumulation in the body
60	*Use with caution* May worsen episodes of fainting in individuals with a history of fainting
61	Avoid long-term use and in patients with certain kidney problems
62	Should not be used for treating side effects of other medications, such as movement side effects of antipsychotic medications
63	Avoid use in patients with heart failure
64	*Use with caution* May cause low sodium levels in blood

Appendix 2

Health History Sheets: What Every Senior Must Have

ELIZABETH ECKSTROM, MD, MPH, MACP

The health history sheet is an invaluable tool for seniors, their families, caregivers, and doctors. Short, concise, and to the point, it assembles in one place a person's doctors, medications, medical health history, and *baseline* cognitive and activity levels. Too often, when an emergency strikes, or even on a day-to-day basis, this vital information cannot be easily retrieved, and decisions are made by healthcare professionals who lack a critical understanding of the "whole" patient and his or her individual history. This can have serious results, ranging from misdiagnoses to ineffective treatment regimes. Many times, these errors set an older person on a trajectory of permanent "step-downs" that *could* have been prevented if only the healthcare team had all the relevant data.

This form can be copied and should be carried at all times by the older person, his or her caregiver, and anyone involved in his or her healthcare, including close family members. It can be laminated for durability and put on the refrigerator for easy retrieval. It can be kept on a flash drive. Each time the patient goes to the doctor, it should be brought in and updated with current health information.

The health history sheet can be thought of as a form with four parts:

Part 1 lists the senior's doctors, their phone numbers, and also a family contact person. It also notes the person's insurance carrier and ID number.

Part 2 is a listing of current medications. These are divided into the times of day the medication is taken (for example, breakfast, mid-morning, lunch, dinner, and bedtime) to make it easier for the patient and caregiver to ensure accuracy of administration. Each medication should have instructions about whether it is to be taken *with or without food* or *with other medications*. For example, calcium (e.g., Tums) should usually be taken by itself, for it can obliterate the effectiveness of other drugs.

Each drug should specify how many milligrams and how many tablets should be taken (e.g., one or two tablets). For some drugs, such as Coumadin, this dose can vary. In these cases, a phone number of the prescribing clinic or pharmacy should be listed next to the drug.

Allergies to medications are also noted at the end of this section.

Part 3 is a succinct summary of a patient's medical history. This is best done together with the patient's primary care provider to ensure accuracy. It should state the patient's age and a brief description of his or her general demeanor. It should accurately record the patient's current cognitive and physical status.

This information is a crucial part of explaining the patient's baseline.

The summary will include a notation of the senior's major medical issues—if he or she has congestive heart failure, diabetes, recurrent urinary tract infections, or mini-strokes, for example. Vision and hearing problems should also be noted, as should other symptoms that trouble the patient on a regular basis (falls, dizziness, low blood pressure, insomnia, depression, etc.). If the patient has been hospitalized, it is helpful to include a sentence or two about the reason for hospitalization and whether the patient has recovered yet.

Part 4 is a table showing a person's "activities of daily living," or "ADLs." This summary of the patient's function is extremely helpful if the person has to go to the emergency department or is hospitalized.

While it takes a little time and effort, conscientiously filling out this form and keeping it updated can make a tremendous difference in your loved one's healthcare management and help him or her to age successfully and safely.

BASELINE and HEALTH HISTORY SHEET

From: The Gift of Caring: Saving Our Parents—and Ourselves—from the Perils of Modern Healthcare Copyright 2015 by Marcy Cottrell Houle, MS and Elizabeth Eckstrom, MD, MPH 2015 (For more information, SEE CHAPTER 27: "The Most Important Word That Can Save Your Loved One's Life" and APPENDIX 2: "Health History Sheets: What Every Senior Must Have") A downloadable version is available at www.giftofcaring.net

SENIOR'S NAME:

Address: _____

Date of Birth: _____ Date of Health History Form: _____

FAMILY CONTACT PERSON: Name; relationship; phone number: _____

_____

DOCTORS:

Primary Care Provider's Name and Phone Number: _____

Specialty Doctor's Name and Phone Number (eg, heart doctor): _____

Additional Specialty Doctor's Name and Phone Number: _____

Insurance: _____

CURRENT MEDICATIONS:

Morning Medications **(indicate if WITH or WITHOUT food):**

NAME and DOSAGE _____

NAME and DOSAGE _____

Lunch:

NAME and DOSAGE _____

NAME and DOSAGE _____

Dinner:

NAME and DOSAGE _____

NAME and DOSAGE _____

Bedtime **(indicate WITH or WITHOUT food):**

NAME and DOSAGE _____

NAME and DOSAGE _____

ALLERGIES:

List known allergies here:

POLST or MOLST: (Physician Orders for Life-Sustaining Treatment): Yes/No?

SENIOR'S CURRENT HEALTH: *BASELINE*

This should be reviewed with the primary care doctor at each visit. It should be a succinct summary of their personal and medical history (including medical issues like heart failure, diabetes, urinary tract infections, dementia, falls, etc.), and should accurately record their current cognitive and physical status. Vision and hearing problems should be noted, as should other symptoms that trouble the patient on a regular basis (falls, dizziness, low blood pressure, insomnia, depression, etc.). If the senior has been hospitalized, include a sentence or two about the reason for hospitalization and how their recovery is going.

SENIOR'S ACTIVITIES OF DAILY LIVING or "ADL's": Date:

Activity	Independent	Needs Some Help	Needs Full Assistance
Dressing			
Bathing			
Toileting			
Eating			
Walking:			
Using a walker?			
Using a cane?			
Transferring			
Cooking			
Using the telephone			
Managing finances			
Managing medications			
Shopping			
Doing laundry			
Doing housekeeping			
Going to places beyond walking distance			
Driving? (yes or no)			
Hearing aid management			

Appendix 3

*Continuity of Care: The Daily Checklist for You,
Your Parent, Your Caregiver, and Your Doctor*

ELIZABETH ECKSTROM, MD, MPH, MACP

*E*very senior who requires the assistance of a caregiver to live comfortably and safely should have "continuity of care" sheets on hand. These forms are vital for two reasons: (1) to provide a daily "health diary" to track subtle changes and (2) to ensure smooth transitions between caregivers. Continuity of care sheets can play an essential role in protecting a loved one's health.

As doctors and nurses are aware, problems routinely occur at "shift change time"—when one caregiver goes off duty and another comes on. Little things can be missed during the handoffs, such as an uneaten meal or signs of confusion—small concerns that, if not noted, can easily begin a slippery downhill slide.

For this reason, keeping a simple form that documents daily activities can reap big benefits. On these forms, caregivers can report when their elder is doing well and what that looks like (giving the healthcare team a good sense of the senior's "baseline") and can note small changes (such as more frequent trips to the bathroom) that family members and clinicians can then review for worrisome patterns. They also allow all caregivers to be *on the same page*—whether they offer help daily or once a week or are family members visiting from far away to give a nearby family caregiver a break. They can be taken to all clinic and hospital visits to furnish the doctor a clear history of the present illness—a tool that can expedite proper treatment.

Continuity of care sheets need not be complicated and can be modified based on the health needs of the senior. Daily sheets should be kept in a folder—or "daybook"—so that a caregiver or family member can easily flip back pages to see what their loved one ate, how much liquid he or she drank, activity level and bowel habits, and general behavior.

This is helpful in providing structure for the patient *and* the person offering care, especially if there are multiple caregivers. For example, if one caregiver cooks meals of meat several days in a row, the next could make fish or a vegetarian main dish. If, under one caregiver's charge, a senior has a busy day with a big outing or lots of visitors, the following day might wisely be a "rest day" to keep the senior from getting worn out. Continuity of care sheets document just that: *continuity*—a factor that can keep our aging loved ones healthier and offer assurance that their needs are being met.

In addition to keeping "continuity of care" sheets, it is often extremely helpful to prepare a "Caregiver's Guide to Mom's (or Dad's) 'Typical' Day." This "schedule" outlines the normal routines for your individual loved one and gives a template for caregivers to follow. It also offers a quick, succinct "biography" of your parent to help caregivers have a personalized understanding. The "Caregiver's Guide to Mom's 'Typical' Day" is especially important if new caregivers are brought in. Additionally, it extends peace of mind to family members who can't be present and want to ensure that their parent's special needs and requests, enjoyments, and preferences are understood and followed.

A sample form for the continuity of care sheet is provided. Also included is the "Caregiver's Guide to Mom's 'Typical' Day" that Marcy made during Margaret's last year of life. Don't be overwhelmed by its complexity. Your care plan can be made much simpler. Plans often start out less involved but require more details as the person ages. Margaret's "Caregiver's Guide" developed over time. It was highly customized and was vital to meeting Margaret's health needs and ensuring her continuing comfort.

Continuity of Care Sheet—*Sample Form*

DATE:

TIME GOT UP: Note hours and quality of sleep pattern

HEARING AID CHECK: Replace battery every Saturday.

SHOWER/BATH:

SHAVE (OR MAKE UP):

ORAL CARE: AM: PM:

NAIL CARE: (hands and feet; attend to every three days):

(OPTIONAL: *Blood pressure:*

                     Temperature:

                     Oxygen:

                     Heart rate:)

BREAKFAST: Time:

                     Foods eaten and amount:

                     Total fluids:

MEDICATIONS GIVEN: (can provide a daily check-off sheet)

EXERCISES:

TOILETING/BOWELS: (if on scheduled toileting, note times here)

LUNCH: Time:

                     Foods eaten and amount:

                     Total fluids:

DINNER: Time:

                     Foods eaten and amount:

                     Total fluids:

DAILY ACTIVITIES AND OUTINGS: List activity and time:

BEHAVIOR: Include notation of any changes or concerns

BEDTIME:

A CAREGIVER'S GUIDE TO MARGARET'S 'TYPICAL' DAY
Who Margaret Is:

Margaret is ninety-three years old. Up until recently, she exhibited good health. Even with her current health concerns and increasing frailty, she still exudes a loving, happy attitude toward life. She is devoted to her family, enjoys her friends, and is a joy to everyone who knows her.

Margaret was married for nearly sixty-one years to Dr. George Cottrell, an orthopedic surgeon, who passed away in April 2000. They enjoyed a happy marriage full of adventures and remained genuinely in love throughout their lives.

George and Margaret built the home where she resides in 1949. She has lived here continually for nearly sixty years and never wants to live anywhere else!

Margaret has three grown daughters with whom she is very close. Ann resides in New Mexico and Karen in Seattle. Marcy and her husband, John, and their two daughters live in town. All her family adores her.

Margaret has always been highly sociable, but today these visits tend to tire her. Her doctor feels that visits should not be for more than two hours. After outings, she will need to rest.

Margaret loves to go shopping (especially at Nordstrom and Chico's), to go to Starbucks for mochas, to visit St. Honore Bakery for croissants, and to take short drives to look at flower gardens or to the beach. She loves to attend church. However, all trips should be limited due to her frailty and will depend on her level of strength that particular day. She also enjoys books on tape, watching movies, and listening to music.

Margaret has always liked to look her best, and it is important that every day she is dressed in clean clothes, has her hair combed, and puts on lipstick and some makeup. She is a refined, intelligent, and caring person who has a generous heart. She has faced all adversity in her life with a great sense of humor, love, and concern for others.

It is our hope that anyone who works with Margaret will realize that she is one of the most special people in the world. Her family will be forever grateful to those caregivers who gently take care of her, encourage her, respect her, and love her. We hope that Margaret will always be treated with great kindness. She is deserving of quality, compassionate care—something she has shown to everyone she has known throughout her life.

(Signed: Marcy Houle)

Margaret's Morning Routine:
   If not up, wake Margaret around 10:00 a.m.

1. *Put in her hearing aid.*
   (Note: Put in a new hearing aid battery every *Saturday*.)
2. Have Margaret do her morning leg exercises.
3. While Margaret is lying down, put on her pants, socks, and shoes (or boots). If Margaret is weak, have her sit in her wheelchair to dress her. If she is strong, sit her up on the side of the bed to finish dressing her. After she is dressed, transfer Margaret to her wheelchair.
4. After Margaret is seated, apply her face cream and put on her makeup, brush and style her hair, put on some jewelry, and apply some perfume. (She likes to look nice!)
5. Take Margaret into the living room and transfer her to her favorite chair.
6. Give her a glass of water with a straw. Put on music. At this time, you can leave her and go to prepare her breakfast.
7. *Before feeding Margaret, be certain to read and understand all feeding instructions.*

   • Margaret has some swallowing issues and her foods must be soft or blended. Absolutely she cannot have nuts, rice, or anything that she could possibly choke on.
   • Feed Margaret small bites of food, and allow plenty of time for her to chew and swallow between bites.
   • When feeding Margaret, put an apron on her. For each meal, serve food on a tray with a cloth napkin. Make a nice food presentation. And make sure she has plenty of water to drink.
   • Margaret bites her cheeks often and needs soft foods and time to eat carefully.
   • Margaret drinks all liquids through a clean straw.

8. *Give Margaret her morning medications.*
9. Do mouth care before and after each meal. Brush her teeth for her, being very careful and gentle, as her gums bleed easily.

After Breakfast:

1. Assist Margaret with her morning exercises.
2. Make Margaret's bed and straighten up her bedroom.
3. Change Margaret's bed on the day of her "bed-bath" and wash, dry, fold, and put away clean sheets.
4. Sometime during the day, write up your information in the *daybook of continuity of care sheets.*

Margaret's Lunchtime Routine: 1:00–2:00 p.m.

1. Give Margaret a snack: either a milkshake with "Ensure" or Jell-O pudding, or a brownie with juice. Make sure she has clean water to drink.

   - *Give lunch medications.*
   - Do mouth care and clean teeth after eating.

2. Margaret's afternoons are generally when she is active. She can go out if her energy allows. Also, during this time, you can read to her, watch a movie with her, or listen to tapes with her.

Late Afternoon: 5:00–7:00 p.m.

1. Do afternoon exercises after a period of rest.

Margaret's Dinner Routine: 7:00 p.m.

1. Offer Margaret a small glass of wine.
2. The dinner routine is much the same as the other meals. Use blended foods.
3. *Give dinner medications.*
4. Do mouth care.

After Dinner: 8:00–9:00 p.m.

1. Offer TV, a movie, or a magazine. Sit and visit with her. Sometimes, after meals, Margaret wants to rest in her chair. This is a good time to clean up the kitchen and do any chores that may need doing.

Bedtime Routine: 9:00–10:00 p.m.

1. During this hour, Margaret is usually ready to go to bed.
2. Call Marcy for her good-night call.
3. Close the bedroom drapes, and turn down Margaret's bed beforehand so that you don't have to leave her alone in her wheelchair or on the side of the bed for the nighttime routine.
4. If Margaret appears weak at night, have her use the commode in the bedroom.
5. Brush and clean Margaret's teeth one final time.
6. Use cleaning cloths to remove her makeup. Put on her night cream.
7. Put on clean Depends if needed.

8. Give Margaret her nighttime pills as she sits in her wheelchair or on the side of the bed.

9. When putting Margaret to bed, be sure to keep her up at the head of her bed as she doesn't like her toes to touch the end of her bed. Also, put socks on her feet, and put a pillow under her legs so that her heels do not rub on the mattress.

10. If it is cool at night, turn on the heater-radiator in her bedroom.

11. Heat up Margaret's neck pad by putting it in the microwave for one to two minutes. Test to make sure it is not too hot.

12. Take out Margaret's hearing aid and open up the battery compartment so that the battery will not run down.

13. Turn out the lights, partially close her door, and leave the hall light on.

14. Lock up the house and turn out the lights except for one in the living room.

15. Hooray! You are done for the day! Thank you!

I tremble with gratitude
for my children and their children
who take pleasure in one another.

At our dinners together, the dead
enter and pass among us
in living love and in memory.

And so the young are taught.

—Wendell Berry